AF228937

MOVE

How Physical Activity Helps Maintain Mental Health

James Roland

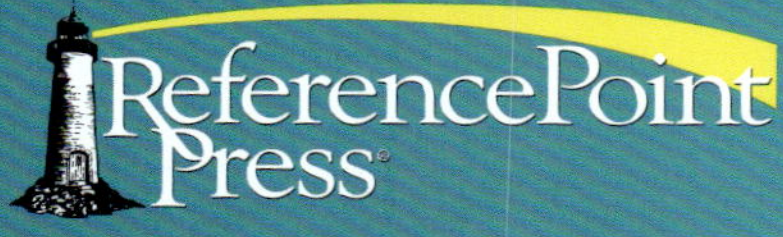

ReferencePoint Press®

San Diego, CA

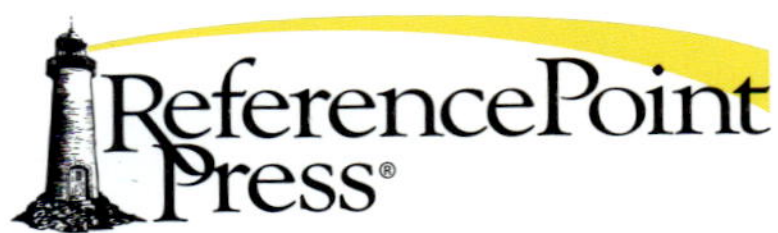

© 2024 ReferencePoint Press, Inc.
Printed in the United States

For more information, contact:
ReferencePoint Press, Inc.
PO Box 27779
San Diego, CA 92198
www.ReferencePointPress.com

LIBRARY OF CONGRESS CATALOGING-IN-PUBLICATION DATA

Names: Roland, James, author.
Title: Move : how physical activity helps maintain mental health / by James Roland.
Description: San Diego, CA : ReferencePoint Press, 2024. | Includes
   bibliographical references and index.
Identifiers: LCCN 2023040298 (print) | LCCN 2023040299 (ebook) | ISBN
   9781678207366 (library binding) | ISBN 9781678207373 (ebook)
Subjects: LCSH: Mental health promotion--Juvenile literature. |
   Exercise--Psychological aspects--Juvenile literature. | Physical
   fitness--Psychological aspects--Juvenile literature.
Classification: LCC RA790.53 .R65 2024 (print) | LCC RA790.53 (ebook) |
   DDC 613.7--dc23/eng/20231002
LC record available at https://lccn.loc.gov/2023040298
LC ebook record available at https://lccn.loc.gov/2023040299

CONTENTS

Stay Active, Feel Better

Think about a group of children playing at recess or splashing around in a swimming pool. Most of the time those kids are smiling and laughing as they run, jump, dive, and keep their bodies in constant motion. It's not just that they are enjoying the games and the company of their friends. Their mood is being buoyed simply by being physically active.

That same kind of mood boost can come from dancing, playing team sports, or just shooting baskets at a nearby playground. You've also probably found yourself feeling a little less stressed just taking a walk around the block, tossing a ball with your dog, or hopping on your bike and riding to a friend's house. You may even forget your troubles for a while doing chores around your home or doing some other type of work that has you up and moving around.

It's not just your imagination. Researchers around the world have compiled countless studies confirming the simple concept that exercise and other types of physical activity help maintain mental health and may help prevent the onset of mental health problems or the relapse of conditions such as depression and anxiety that have already been treated. The connection between physical activity and better mental health is undeniable. "Studies suggest that physical exercise may help ward off mental health problems before they start. Research also shows exercise can improve the symptoms of many existing mental illnesses,"[1] mental health counselor Katharina Star wrote in an article for the website Verywell Mind.

Movement Helps Manage Stress

As a coping mechanism, physical activity can help young people—and anyone, really—deal with stress and climb out of periods of emotional and psychological struggle. In Massachusetts, Taunton High School student Caitlin Lincoln joined several fellow students in giving a TED talk about teen mental health in the spring of 2022. She said she found that regular exercise and journaling helped her cope with an especially difficult time in her life—the stress of the early COVID-19 lockdowns and limits on school activities. "Exercise can improve your health physically and mentally,"[2] she said, adding that she had initially avoided healthy coping mechanisms before discovering the benefits of being active.

You don't even need to work up a sweat or put in hours of activity each day to start reaping the emotional and psychological benefits of movement, according to Jeremy Whitworth, executive director of Trails Carolina, a wilderness therapy program for teens. "Studies have shown that the health benefits of exercise in teens can significantly improve depression or anxiety," he wrote on the Trails Carolina website. "Even just getting 30 minutes of exercise a few times a week can improve overall mood. Exercising with an anxiety disorder can actually help reduce symptoms in teens and allow them to calm down."[3]

> "Even just getting 30 minutes of exercise a few times a week can improve overall mood."[3]
>
> —Jeremy Whitworth, executive director of Trails Carolina

For example, a 2023 Finnish study of adolescents found that engaging in leisure-time physical activities of just thirty minutes a week was associated with significantly lower risks of having symptoms of chronic stress, depression, or anxiety. The study's findings, published in the *Scandinavian Journal of Medicine &*

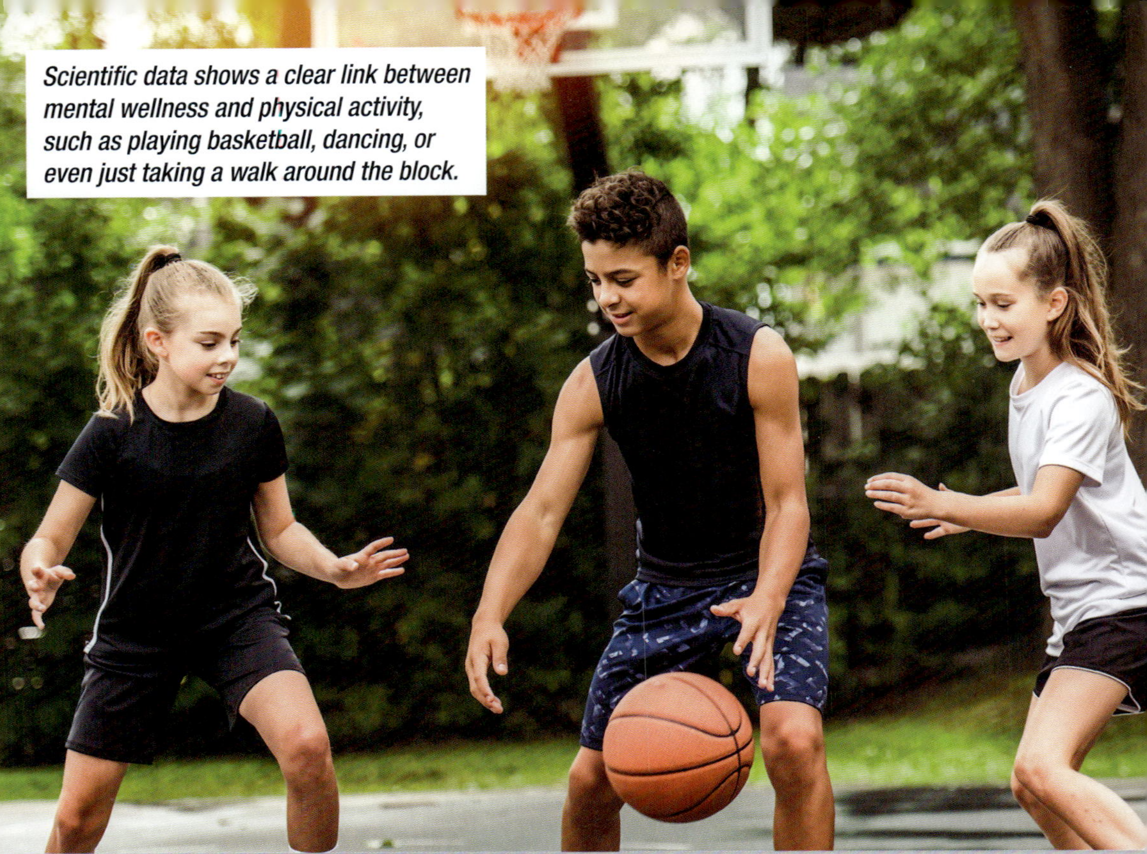

Science in Sports, also note that the youths who were the most physically active tended to have the lowest odds of mental health symptoms compared with their peers who weren't active.

Brain Benefits of Exercise

Physical activity bolsters good mental health for several reasons, including exercise-induced changes in brain chemistry and circulation, as well as other benefits related to self-confidence, socialization, and stress relief. And while various activities each offer their own sets of mental health advantages—running and swimming help clear your mind, while team sports promote a sense of purpose and belonging—physical activity of any kind will improve your mood and your overall health. "Pick something you can sustain over time," suggests Michael Craig Miller, assistant professor of psychiatry at Harvard Medical School. "The key is to make it something you like and something that you'll want to keep doing."[4] Recruit your friends and family members to join you. The socialization associated with certain activities delivers mental health boosts, too.

Like those little kids running around the playground or jumping into a swimming pool, you can enjoy physical activity for the simple pleasure it provides, without focusing on the benefits to mental health or physical fitness. But when you do think about how to overcome emotional or psychological challenges or perhaps steer clear of them in the first place, know that moving your body is about the simplest, least-expensive way to go about it.

CHAPTER ONE

The Mind–Body Connection

Every day Florida high school senior Beatrice Shen carries the stress that inevitably comes with juggling a challenging academic load, extracurricular activities, and other responsibilities. But the Palm Harbor University High School student found a way to handle those pressures by enrolling in a dance studio not far from her home. "I feel like when I dance, I just forget about everything else that's going on and I'm very in the moment," she said in an interview with Bay News 9, a local TV news station, calling dance "a good stress coping mechanism for me."[5]

Shen is such a believer in dance's ability to help people de-stress that she organized a dance program for other kids and to raise money and awareness for youth mental health in her community. Dance and other aerobic exercises can help reduce stress and improve mood in a few different ways. Physical activity, for example, reduces levels of cortisol, a hormone produced in the adrenal glands but activated by the brain in response to stress or fear. Under normal conditions, cortisol helps the brain and body deal with fear or stress, but when elevated for lengthy periods, it can contribute to anxiety and depression. "Exercise has a dramatic antidepressive effect," says David J. Linden, a professor of neuroscience at the Johns Hopkins University School of Medicine. "It blunts the brain's response to physical and emotional stress."[6]

By lowering the body's stress levels, you're not just feeling more relaxed; you're also supporting your immune system, which also helps keep you physically healthy. And that's just one of many ways the health of your mind and body are intertwined. You may not have thought about it that way but stop and consider all the times you've had strong emotions that had corresponding physical symptoms. That nervousness before a big test may have given you an uneasy feeling in your stomach. Perhaps being scared in a carnival haunted house got your heart racing. Or maybe being angry caused the muscles in the back of your neck and scalp to tense up, leading to a headache.

Better Mood, Better Health

Positive moods also improve bodily health. Feeling happy and relaxed eases muscle tension. People often say they feel "lighter" during joyous moments, a sensation likely related to the release of hormones such as dopamine and serotonin—both of which are associated with positive moods. The rush and excitement of winning a sports championship can seem to ease the physical pain of an injury, at least for a little while. Simply laughing supports cardiovascular health. "Laughter increases oxygen intake and helps regulate heart rate and breathing through the relaxation response that often follows in the wake of a laugh,"[7] says Scott Janssen, a clinical social worker at the University of North Carolina.

But the mind-body connection doesn't just affect a moment here or there. Long-term and serious health concerns also demonstrate how your emotions are tied to physical health. For example, while depression can trigger temporary headaches, digestive problems, and bouts of fatigue, it's also associated with increased risks of cancer and heart disease. Likewise, people with chronic diseases or severe injuries are at higher risk for mental health challenges like depression, anxiety, loneliness, and other issues.

One reason that people with depression are at higher risk for heart disease or cancer is that depression can often prevent people from seeing a doctor regularly and taking good care of themselves. For example, those who suffer from depression might engage in poor behaviors such as unhealthy eating, not getting enough sleep, and in many cases, not being active enough to keep the brain and body fit.

Fortunately, some of the same behaviors that promote a healthy mood do the same for a healthy body. A good diet, for example, can nourish your muscles and organs while also fueling a positive outlook and improving brain functions. Getting enough sleep is just as crucial as getting enough good nutrition to support your overall well-being. And, as Shen and countless other active individuals will attest, keeping your body moving not only energizes and strengthens the body, it also allows you to relax and better manage the mental challenges you face in school, at home, and elsewhere.

The more you understand how physical activity triggers so many healthy responses in the body—including those that affect

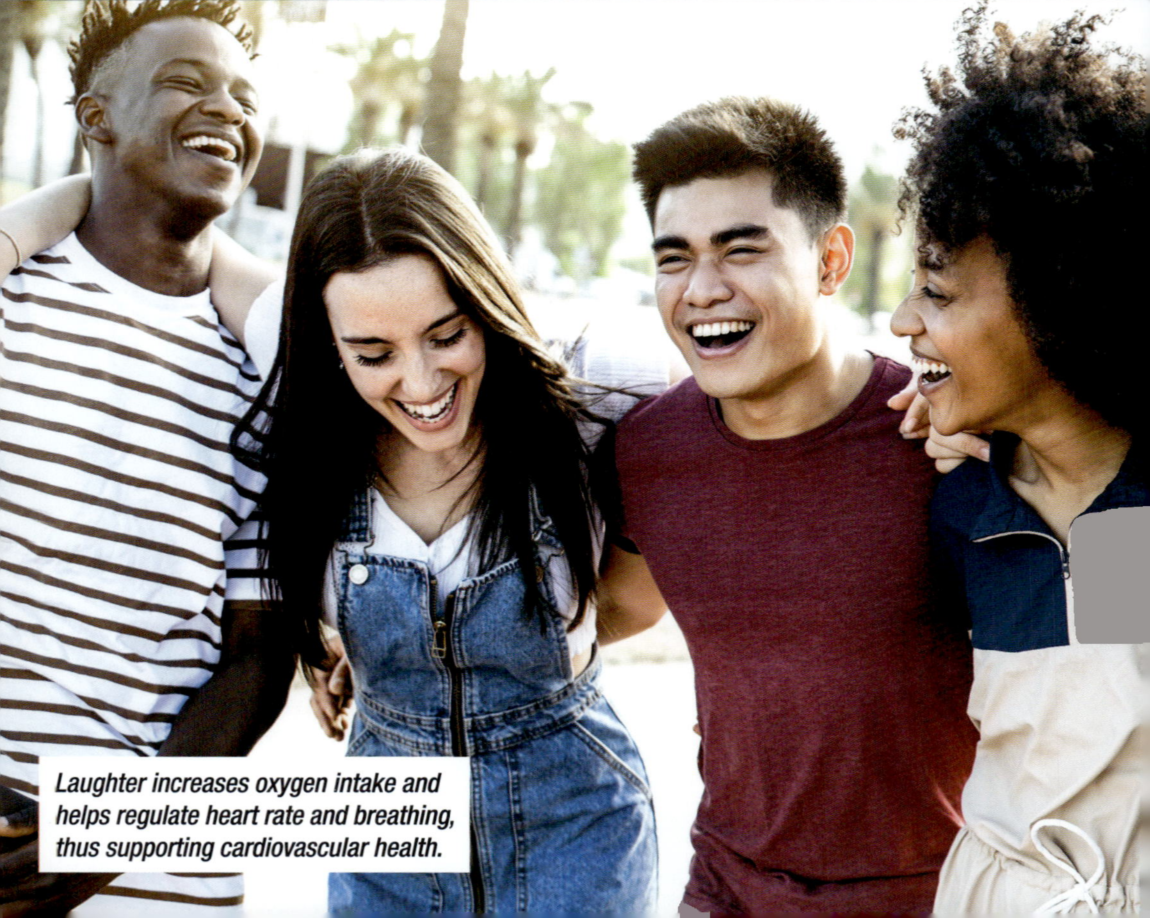

Laughter increases oxygen intake and helps regulate heart rate and breathing, thus supporting cardiovascular health.

your mental health—the more motivated you might be to get up and get moving. Similarly, the more aware you are of how a lack of physical activity can result in a range of physical and mental difficulties, the more inspired you can be to put yourself on a healthier track.

The Risks of Too Much Sitting

Sometimes plopping yourself down in a comfy chair after a long day is just what you need to relax your mind and body. Sitting for too long, however, is not what your mind and body need. In fact, several studies in recent years have found that people who sit for extended periods of time are at higher risk for depression and have a harder time paying attention and thinking clearly.

British psychiatrist Aaron Kandola led a study of kids aged twelve, fourteen, and sixteen and found that those who spent the most time sitting throughout the week had far more symptoms of depression compared with their peers who spent the most time being physically active. His research echoed similar findings of other studies that looked at the association between a sedentary lifestyle and low mood. "It is great to exercise and play sports," he said in a 2021 article on the Science News Explores website. "But anything you can do to avoid sitting for too long at once will help with mood, stress and thinking clearly. Interestingly, the more you sit down, the more tired you tend to feel, too."[8]

When the COVID-19 pandemic upended normal activities in 2020 and kept people away from school, work, and each other, researchers set out to assess how such abrupt changes might affect mental health. A team of researchers from Iowa State University found that as sitting time and screen time increased, so did symptoms of loneliness, anxiety, and depression. "Sitting is a sneaky behavior," says Jacob Meyer, assistant professor of kinesiology (the study of how the body moves) at Iowa State University and the study's lead researcher. "It's something we do all the time without thinking about it."[9]

What Is Mental Health?

Mental health refers to a person's emotional and psychological well-being. It influences how you feel and, to a great extent, how you think and act. Your mental health affects how you relate to the people around you and how you handle stress and any challenges you face. Mental health is not always stable; sometimes it changes from day to day or slowly over time. If you're dealing with a serious family crisis, for example, you may also experience poor mental health. But if that crisis ends with a positive outcome, your mental health may improve. Mental health problems can develop due to biological factors, such as chemical imbalances in the brain, or due to environmental factors, such as trauma. For many people a mental health disorder, such as depression or anxiety, can take a long time and many hours of therapy to resolve. Milder mental health challenges may be met with a combination of healthy lifestyle changes and professional counseling. While you can't always prevent the onset of a mental health challenge, you can lower your risk by exercising, eating right, getting enough sleep, and learning ways to manage stress.

Meyer's follow-up research found that as people adjusted to pandemic-related lockdowns and more time at home by becoming more active, their self-reported symptoms of anxiety and depression lessened. Researchers are still trying to understand why sedentary behavior is so strongly associated with anxiety, depression, and low mood, but it may have something to do with missing out on the many positive mental health benefits of being physically active.

What Happens When You Move

Physical activity stimulates many positive changes in your brain and the rest of your body. As your heart rate increases due to physical exertion, so does blood flow to the brain. An increase in oxygen and other nutrients in the bloodstream nourishes existing brain cells (neurons) and spurs the formation of new brain cells. This process, called neurogenesis, helps support thinking skills, memory, and other brain functions throughout your life. "Right now, there is no substitute for regular exercise to help with neurogenesis,"[10] says Rudolph Tanzi, a world-renowned brain function researcher and codirector of the McCance Center for Brain Health at Massachusetts General Hospital in Boston.

Exercise-fueled new brain cells counteract depression's negative influence on the size and activity of certain brain regions associated with mood. "In people who are depressed, neuroscientists have noticed that the hippocampus in the brain—the region that helps regulate mood—is smaller. Exercise supports nerve cell growth in the hippocampus, improving nerve cell connections, which helps relieve depression,"[11] says Michael Craig Miller, assistant professor of psychiatry at Harvard Medical School.

One of the building blocks of new neurons is a protein called brain-derived neurotrophic factor (BDNF). It not only promotes the growth of new neurons, it also protects existing ones, fostering better communication between brain cells and keeping the circuitry in our brains running smoothly. "Evidence suggests that aerobic exercise can increase molecules in the brain, such as BDNF,"[12] says Lindsey Wooliscroft, assistant

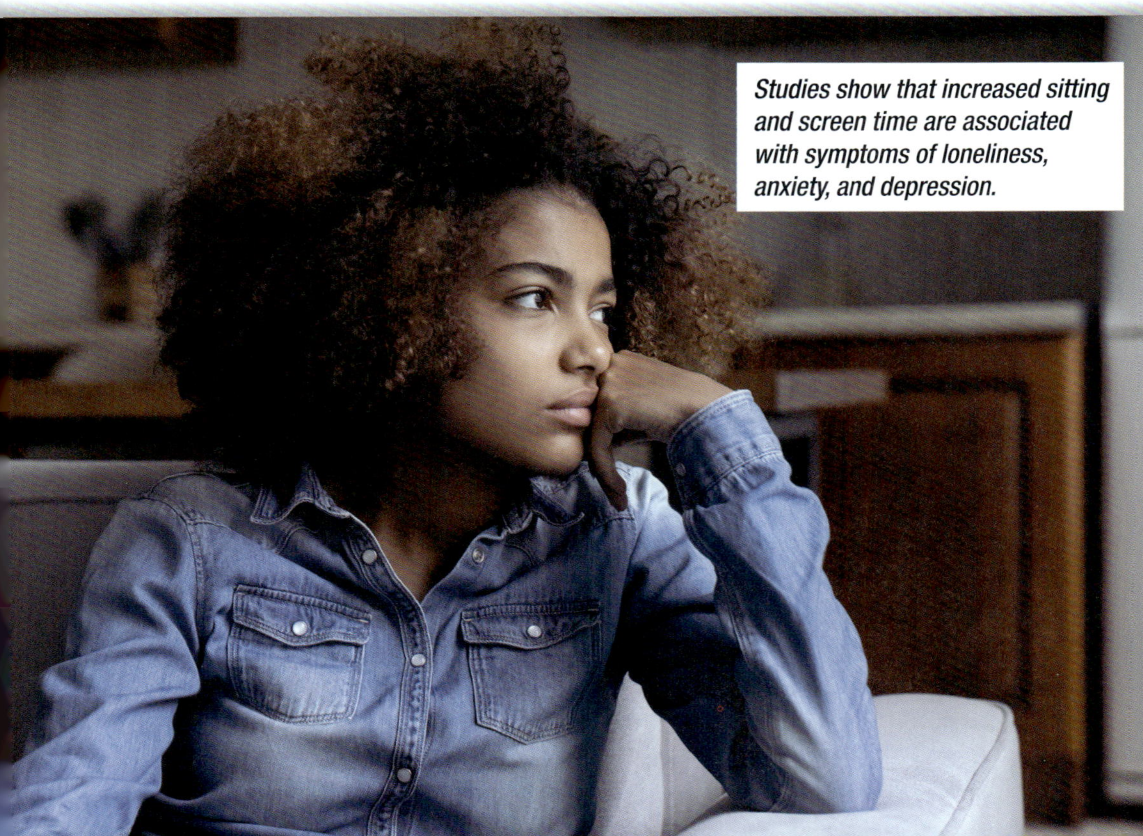

Studies show that increased sitting and screen time are associated with symptoms of loneliness, anxiety, and depression.

professor of neurology at Oregon Health & Science University. She adds that low levels of BDNF are associated with serious neurological disorders, such as Alzheimer's disease and Parkinson's disease, as well as depression and other types of mental illness.

Aerobic exercise also increases blood flow to the brain. In an essay about exercise and brain function published in *Scientific American*, Justin Rhodes, an associate professor of psychology at the University of Illinois, Urbana-Champaign, wrote, "More blood flow means more energy and oxygen, which makes our brains perform better."[13] He explained that exercise is also helpful in enhancing how well you learn new things and recall information you've already learned. He also wrote that increased circulation to the brain may also improve how well we assess risks and make decisions, noting that our ancestors ran from predators or toward prey, and that physical activity probably helped them make a lot of decisions that increased their chances of survival.

A Boost to Energy and Overall Well-Being

Being able to think more clearly, concentrate for longer periods of time, make thoughtful decisions, and remember information with greater detail can translate to successful classroom achievement, better problem-solving skills, and the ability to express yourself more clearly. The act of running or jogging, for example, allows you to focus on your breathing and on the simple act of putting one foot in front of the other. It helps set aside other distractions in your mind and really lets you take control of your thought processes. "People that engage in journeys of increased physical activity often learn how to set and achieve goals, how to problem solve, how to plan and organize their activities," says Rhonda Merwin, an associate professor of psychiatry and behavioral sciences at Duke University. "They learn how to self-monitor and track their own behavior and regulate their internal experiences with mindful awareness of the breath."[14]

Don't Forget to Eat Right

Moving more helps maintain mental and physical health, but so does a balanced diet. Make sure you fuel up with a diet rich in fruits, vegetables, whole grains, and lean proteins. Be aware that processed foods and those with added sugars sap your energy and depress your mood. For many people, eating healthier means making simple food swaps: a bowl of berries for dessert instead of cookies, for example. If you're a very active person, such as a swimmer or runner, your calorie needs will probably be higher than those of people who are sedentary. If you lift weights and are trying to build muscle, you may need more protein than the average person. And if you are obese, a condition that affects about one in five teens in the United States, you may want to work with a dietitian or nutritionist to help map out an eating strategy that helps you achieve and maintain a healthy weight. Your doctor may be able to write a prescription for a dietitian's services. Even if you aren't obese, you may benefit from talking with an expert about how to eat right for your health and activity level.

Regular exercise also gives you more energy and helps keep you looking and feeling fit. All these benefits can enhance your self-esteem and give you more confidence. Exercise also triggers the release of chemicals such as dopamine and endorphins, both of which boost mood. When a long, intense workout leads to extremely high levels of endorphins, the effect is sometimes referred to as a "runner's high," but other aerobic workouts can produce similar good feelings.

Endorphins also provide special benefits for people who exercise together. A 2016 study in the journal *Adaptive Human Behavior and Physiology* suggests that a group of dancers dancing in synchrony experience a release of endorphins that fosters a sense of belonging and even increases their pain threshold. Separate studies of rowers and other athletes working in synchrony have demonstrated similar results. Psychologist Kelly McGonigal, author of *The Joy of Movement*, explains:

> Whoever you move with, whether it's a walking group or maybe a group class, because of the way exercise alters our brain chemistry and outlook, you start to feel a true

sense of connection with the people that you're moving with. It's why people will talk about people who they work out with as their "fitness fam." Because it really does give us a sense of belonging, it helps build relationships that can be true friendships and sources of support.[15]

Exercise and Sleep

While regular physical activity is essential for good mental health, you also need to stop and rest every day. You may have noticed that at the end of an especially active day, you often sleep a little better than usual. Sometimes that good night's sleep is due to physical exhaustion. But regular exercise also helps set your circadian rhythms—the body's sleep-wake cycle that can ensure you get enough quality sleep. "We have solid evidence that exercise does, in fact, help you fall asleep more quickly and improves sleep quality," says Dr. Charlene Gamaldo, medical director of the Johns Hopkins Center for Sleep in Maryland. "But there's still some debate as to what time of day you should exercise. I encourage people to listen to their bodies to see how well they sleep in response to when they work out."[16]

Many sleep experts recommend against workouts too close to bedtime, however. Aerobic exercise triggers the release of endorphins that can stimulate brain activity that gets in the way of falling asleep. Exercise also increases core body temperature, and even a slight bump in temperature can signal the body that it's time to be awake and alert. Once your core body temperature starts to come down, it's easier to fall asleep. If possible, try to do most of your exercise—especially aerobic, vigorous activity—at least a couple of hours before bedtime. If that doesn't fit your schedule, or your workouts don't seem to affect your ability to fall asleep and sleep well through the night, then do

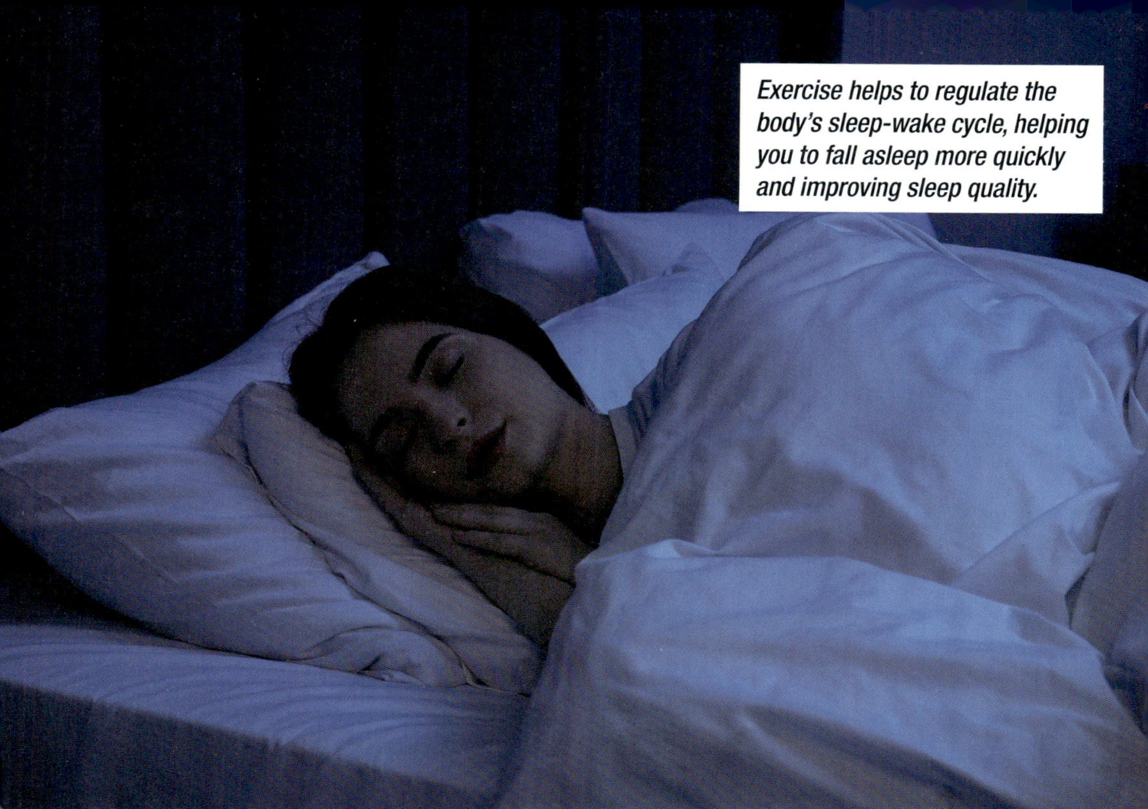

what works best for you. "Know your body and know yourself," Gamaldo says. "Doctors definitely want you to exercise, but when you do it is not scripted."[17]

Sleep is an essential component of mental health. Without sufficient sleep on a consistent basis, you can become irritable, feel moody, and have trouble concentrating and making decisions. When you're young, getting enough sleep is crucial for brain development and brain functions, like recalling information and paying attention. Over time, insufficient sleep can be a risk factor for depression and anxiety. Alex Agostini, a researcher at the University of South Australia, has studied how sleep is crucial for maintaining mental health, but its importance is too often overlooked—especially among teenagers. She says:

> Getting enough sleep is important for all of us—it helps our physical and mental health, boosts our immunity, and ensures we can function well on a daily basis. But for teenagers, sleep is especially critical because they're at an age

where they're going through a whole range of physical, social, and developmental changes, all of which depend on enough sleep.

Research shows that teenagers need at least eight hours of sleep each night. Without this, they're less able to deal with stressors, such as bullying or social pressures, and run the risk of developing behavioural problems, as well as anxiety and depression.[18]

If you have trouble falling asleep or you wake up throughout the night, talk with a parent or guardian or with a doctor. The solution may be something as simple as sticking to a consistent sleep schedule or turning off your phone and other electronic screens an hour before bedtime. If the problem is more complicated or not easily solved by adjusting your sleep routine, you may need to see a sleep specialist for more assistance.

CHAPTER TWO

Movement and Mental Health

The COVID-19 pandemic meant countless high school students around the United States would be taking classes online and missing out on sports, theater, proms, and just hanging out together in person. Alex Ramirez, the soccer coach at Riverside High School in Durham, North Carolina, worried that his players' mental health would suffer without the routine of practices and the camaraderie of teammates. He was right—his players regularly confided in him how depressed and isolated they felt.

So in the winter of 2020–2021, when an abbreviated soccer season began, Ramirez's players once again found joy, relief, and more on the soccer pitch. Junior Reese Compton said playing soccer served as an escape from the monotony of online school and other COVID-19-related challenges in his life, like missing out on events and activities that usually fill the high school calendar. "It gave me something to focus on that I could do to distract myself from all the bad things going on,"[19] he told his school newspaper, the *Pirate's Hook*. Teammate Logan Armstrong agreed. "It improved my mental health, since I had something to do after school and look forward to, too,"[20] he told the school newspaper.

Sports and other physical activities can improve mood, even without something as serious as a public health crisis hanging overhead. Bursts of physical activity can certainly provide immediate and short-term mood-elevating benefits. But over time, regular exercise can often help keep symptoms of depression and anxiety at bay and become an effective part of your treatment if you do struggle with these or other mood disorders. "Moderate activity of any kind, getting out and doing something, is associated with improvements, lower levels of depressive symptoms, lower levels of anxiety, better well-being,"[21] says Elaine McMahon, a public health researcher in Ireland, who led a study of exercise's effects on mental health involving more than eleven thousand teenagers in ten countries.

Plenty of people who experience stress are aware of how effective movement can be in helping them relax, but too few actually exercise to help overcome their stress. The Anxiety and Depression Association of America reports that only about 14 percent of the people who acknowledge experiencing stress or anxiety daily turn to exercise to help them cope. That's the same percentage of people who said they turned to food as their way of dealing with stress. You may not think of physical activity as a type of medicine to treat stress or a mental health disorder or lower your risk of developing such a problem, but the evidence is clear that even without a prescription, exercise is just what the doctor ordered.

Exercise Protects Against Depression

The image you might have of depression treatment is someone sitting on a couch talking with a therapist or taking an antidepressant medication. But there is a growing body of research to suggest that a key way to cope with depression is to get off the couch and get moving. In one of the largest examinations of exercise as a treatment for depression, published in the summer of 2023 in the *British Journal of Sports Medicine*, German researchers reviewed more than forty studies and found that nearly any type of physical activity, even just walking a few days a week, reduces depression symptoms. "Something is better than nothing,"[22] says lead researcher Andreas Heissel, noting that people shouldn't as-

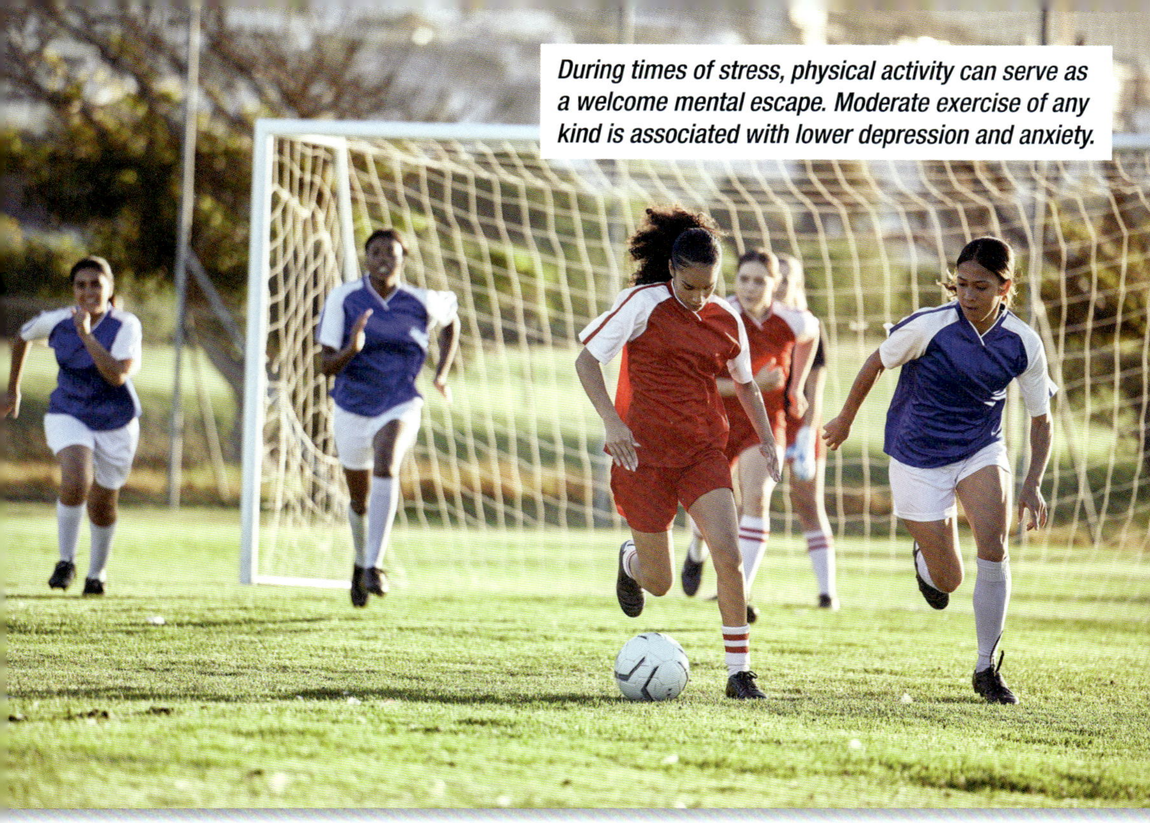

sume that only strenuous exercise performed for hours at a time can offer any benefits.

While physical activity may help if you are already experiencing depression, exercise may also help prevent the onset of depression. A Harvard study found that running for fifteen minutes a day or walking for an hour a day may help reduce the risk of depression onset by 26 percent.

It's worth noting that people who are physically active aren't immune to conditions such as depression. Depression is a condition that can run in families and can develop due to an imbalance of brain chemicals, childhood trauma, and many other causes beyond an individual's control. You can exercise, eat right, and make every smart, healthy decision possible and still be faced with depression, anxiety, or some other type of mental illness.

To demonstrate how depression can affect anyone, successful athletes have become more open in recent years about how depression and other mental health disorders have added to the challenges of their sporting pursuits as well as how physical

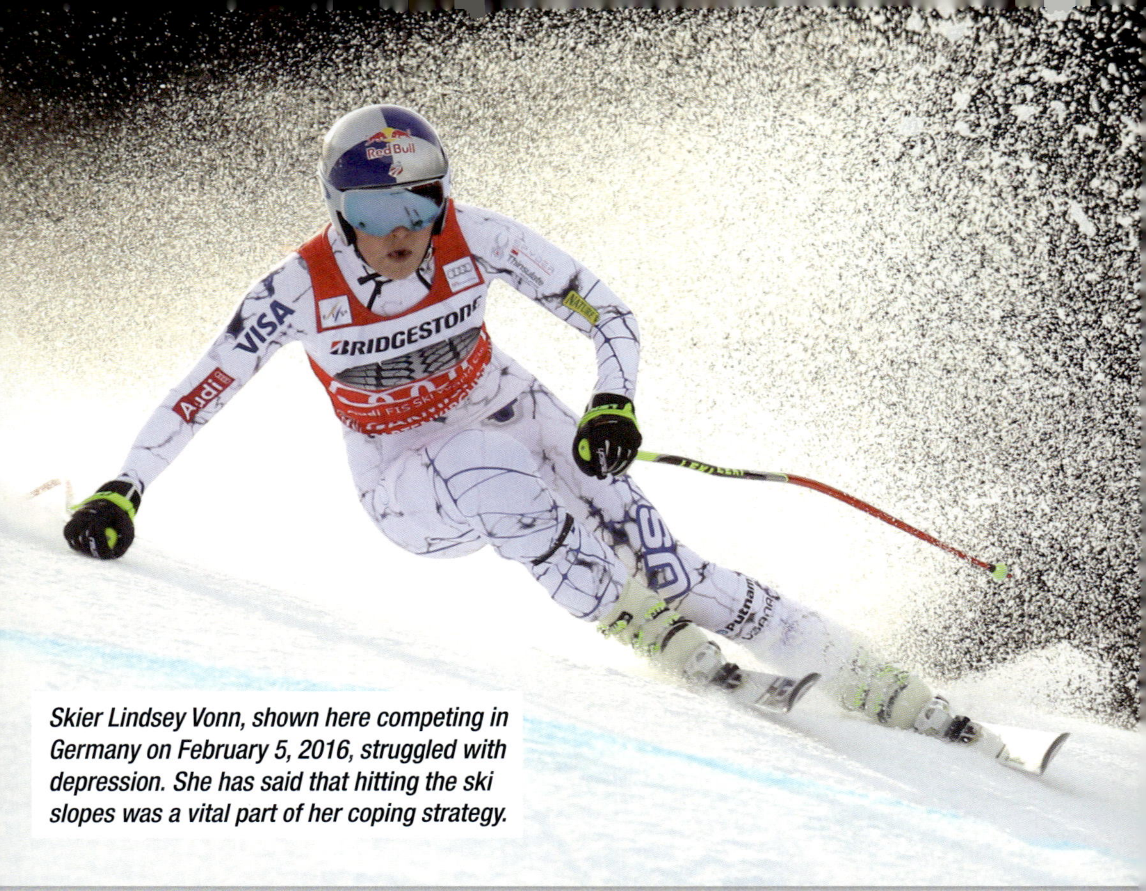

Skier Lindsey Vonn, shown here competing in Germany on February 5, 2016, struggled with depression. She has said that hitting the ski slopes was a vital part of her coping strategy.

activity helped them manage their mental health. Olympic gold medal skier Lindsey Vonn, for example, told CNBC in 2021 that she had struggled with depression since her teenage years. And though losing races and getting injured often made her depressive symptoms worse, she found that getting back on the slopes was a vital part of her coping strategy. "No matter how depressed I got, skiing always made me happy,"[23] she said.

Sweat Your Stress Away

Exercise isn't just helpful in easing symptoms of depression or lowering your risk of developing a mental health disorder. Being physically active is also one of the most effective ways to relieve stress and clear your head. Whether you're playing a sport that requires a lot of moment-to-moment decision-making and strategy or you're casually swimming laps in a pool, your brain has a way of focusing on the movement of your muscles and limbs, your breathing, and the next milestone. As a result, you can essentially set aside the big worries and stresses in your life or the little inconveniences and frustrations that might otherwise occupy your mind—at least for a little while.

In California, Cuesta College soccer player Emma Nushi always relied on her sport as a welcome break from whatever stress she was experiencing. In a column for her college newspaper, the *Cuestonian*, she wrote:

No matter what I had going on in my life, whether it was stress at home or at school, soccer was always there and it was always the same. It was something I could count on. Even if I was having the worst day of all time, for two hours in the afternoon, I would get to go to practice where everything made sense to me and for a little while, nothing else existed. For as long as I can remember, soccer has been the thing that I cling to when nothing else makes sense.[24]

But you don't have to play on an organized sports team to enjoy the stress-reducing benefits of physical activity. You can turn your focus away from your troubles and toward dance, martial arts, surfing, skating, or myriad other activities to boost your mental health and reduce your stress levels. You can even pedal your stress away on your bicycle. "Our research shows that kids who get out for a bike ride at least once a week report higher levels of mental well-being,"[25] says cognitive scientist Esther Walker, research program manager at Outride, a nonprofit organization that conducts cycling research and supports programming for youth.

Managing stress is important, not just so you can feel more relaxed but also because stress can sap your energy and make it harder to focus and do your work. Over time, stress can lead

Get Outside When You Can

The weather and your surroundings can often conspire to keep you indoors, but if you get the chance to get out in the fresh air, it's worth it. Numerous studies in recent years have shown the mental health benefits of being out in nature, including reduced levels of loneliness, stress, anxiety, and depression and improvements in focus and feelings of calmness. Time spent in nature is also associated with improved memory and thinking skills. "There is mounting evidence, from dozens and dozens of researchers, that nature has benefits for both physical and psychological human wellbeing," says Lisa Nisbet, a psychologist at Trent University in Canada and a researcher who studies humans' relationship with nature. "You can boost your mood just by walking in nature, even in urban nature. And the sense of connection you have with the natural world seems to contribute to happiness even when you're not physically immersed in nature."

Quoted in Kirsten Weir, "Nurtured by Nature," American Psychological Association, April 1, 2020. www.apa.org.

to physical problems like heart disease and high blood pressure, as well as mental health challenges like depression and anxiety. Stress can also lead to unhealthy ways of trying to cope, such as overeating or eating unhealthy foods, getting too little sleep, turning to alcohol or drugs, or engaging in other reckless or dangerous behaviors. Conversely, bringing down your stress levels can give your self-esteem a big boost.

Exercise and Self-Esteem

That's important because your self-esteem can take hits from all sides: social media and mass media, family, classmates, and even friends who might mean well but still say things that can have you questioning everything from the way you look and dress to the way you behave and the things you say. But one way to quietly but effectively boost your self-confidence is through exercise and sports. Incremental improvements in your skills—how much weight you can lift, for example—or other areas of fitness can go a long way toward enhancing how you view yourself. "Over time, you get better at something you're doing, and you develop a sense of mastery and feeling that you're getting stronger," says

James Whitworth, a doctoral research fellow in the Biobehavioral Resistance Training Lab at Columbia University's Teachers College in New York City. "It helps your confidence, and that gives you a boost in self-esteem."[26]

When you feel better about yourself and your health or fitness, you may be more confident in other areas of your life. You may become more outgoing and less shy. You may have more confidence in the classroom or in social situations. But sometimes people need a little extra boost to feel that they're really making progress.

Step counters or pedometers are everywhere, from smartwatches and smartphones to little devices clipped to a belt or even built into sneakers. One reason why pedometers are so popular is that they provide a running tally of the steps you've taken. You can set a specific number of steps for the day or for a workout and see whether you reached your goal. Hitting your target offers immediate satisfaction and a sense of accomplishment. While taking ten thousand steps per day has become a popular target, it's important not to get too caught up in counting steps; instead, focus on the idea that accumulating a lot of steps per day can benefit your physical fitness and your mental well-being. "Don't obsess about the number of steps, but try to go for a walk every day," says David Geier, an orthopedic surgeon and sports medicine specialist in South Carolina. "Hopefully it will become a habit and encourage you to become active in other ways in your life."[27]

The same is true for other exercise and sports goals. You don't want to set unrealistic goals (which can lead to disappointment and frustration) or become so focused on setting new goals that you don't appreciate the successes along the way. Take time to recognize that achieving success in any activity enhances your motivation to remain active and brings with it rewards that increase confidence and self-esteem.

The key is to have short-term achievable goals and targets as well as more ambitious milestones you're trying to reach. If you want to use steps as an easy way to measure your activity and monitor your progress, start with a daily goal of three thousand steps, for example, and build up from there. Likewise, you might want to aim for an hour of exercise a day, but at the beginning start with a ten-minute goal. Simply noting your increased activity levels over the course of a week or month will motivate you to keep going and will remind you that you are capable of setting and reaching goals—important features of self-confidence.

Socializing and Exercising

Walking or riding your skateboard around your neighborhood on your own may be the kind of "alone time" everyone needs from time to time. But humans are social creatures and need interpersonal interactions to survive. Playing team sports or engaging in other physical activities with friends, classmates, family members, and even people you don't know increases your social interactions—a cornerstone of good mental health. Regular social interaction is also a critical component of healthy thinking skills for people of all ages.

Exercising with others can help keep you from feeling lonely and can boost your self-worth. Participating in group activities also enhances your feelings of belonging and provides a sense of purpose, both of which support optimal mental health. "Studies have shown that the No. 1 reason most adults start and continue an exercise program is the social component," University of Texas exercise physiologist Carol Harrison told CNN in 2022. "Kids are the same."[28]

While exercise in just about any form supports better mental health, you may find additional benefits by incorporating team sports or group activities into your overall activity regimen. Psychologist and researcher Susan Pinker said in a 2022 article in Virginia Tech's student newspaper *Collegiate Times*:

Face-to-face contact releases a whole cascade of neurotransmitters [chemical messengers], and like a vaccine,
they protect you now in the present and well into the future.
So simply making eye contact with somebody, shaking
hands, giving somebody a high-five is enough to release
oxytocin, which increases your level of trust and it lowers
your cortisol levels. So it lowers your stress. And dopamine
is generated, which gives us a little high and it kills pain.[29]

Training for Academic Success

Along with its many mood-enhancing benefits, regular physical
activity can also help you develop discipline, focus, motivation,
and balance in your life. These qualities can help in school, at
work, at home, or in any environment in which your time, energy,
and attention are challenged. Californian Dean Carpentier, a mem-
ber of the Huntington Beach High School baseball team, credits
the self-discipline and focus he acquired in baseball for helping
him succeed in the classroom. He says he doesn't feel the same
kind of academic pressure many of his peers do because he has

had to make time for school and baseball for years. "There's a discipline I have learned where balancing both has become easy but that's not pressure,"[30] he told *Slick*, his high school's student magazine.

Success in athletics or other pursuits such as performing arts can also be especially important if you struggle academically. Knowing you can achieve in one area can give you the confidence to keep trying elsewhere. And if you need a certain grade point average to be eligible to participate in certain school activities, your success on the ball field or the stage may provide enough motivation to work toward success in the classroom.

In addition to providing an outlet for academic pressure or motivation to work harder in the classroom, regular exercise can also translate to improved levels of concentration and focus in school and elsewhere. Exercise can even help improve attention among students with challenges such as attention-deficit/hyperactivity

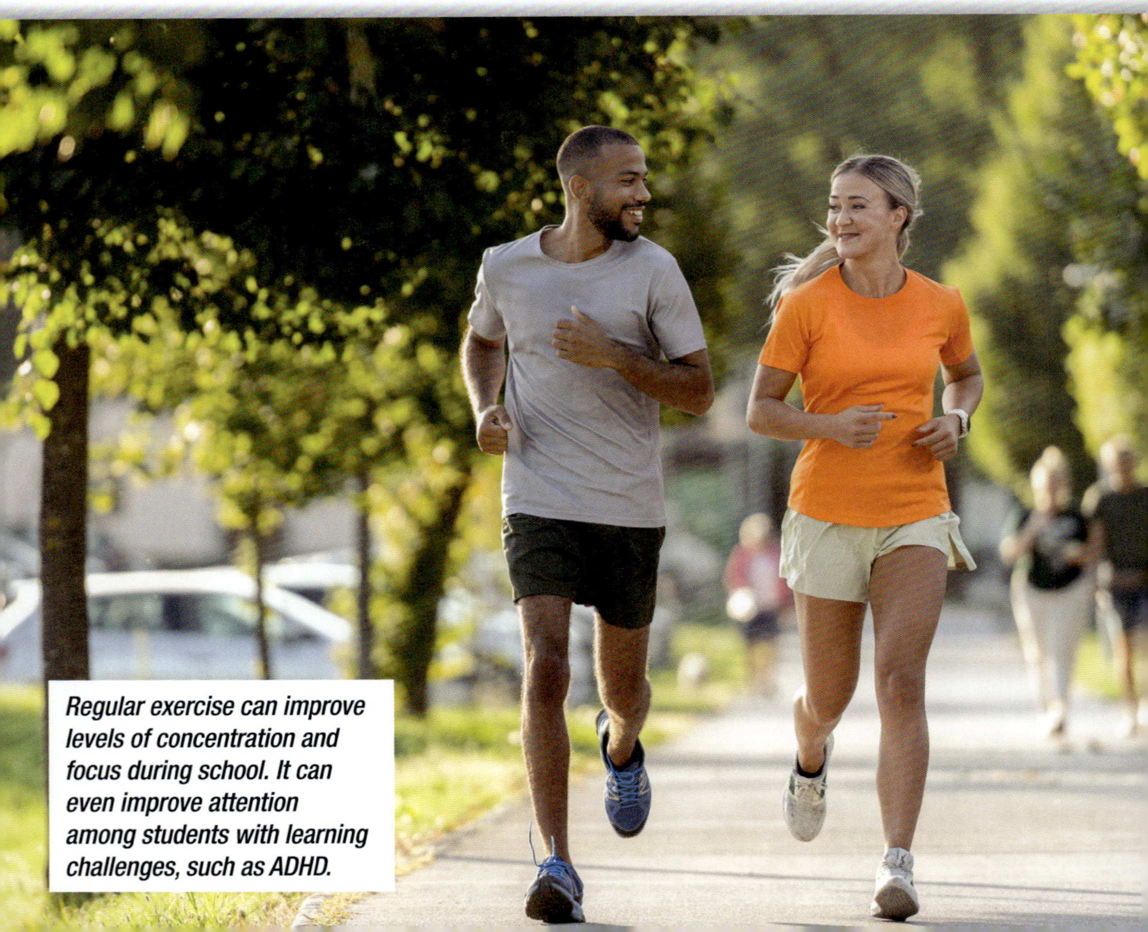

Regular exercise can improve levels of concentration and focus during school. It can even improve attention among students with learning challenges, such as ADHD.

disorder (ADHD). Jackson, a twenty-one-year-old college student who was diagnosed with ADHD in elementary school, found that he was able to stop taking the ADHD drug Ritalin after he took up running. "When I started exercising, I suddenly was able to concentrate on things that were important to me," he says. "There's never been any question in my mind that exercise is related to concentration. Once I made this huge life change, and committed to exercise, it was very clear to me that things started to change in my life."[31]

Jackson's physician, John Ratey, notes that while many people with ADHD will still need medication if they exercise regularly, it's possible that some may be able to go off it completely or at least reduce their dosage. He explains that exercise increases levels of dopamine and norepinephrine, which are neurotransmitters in the brain that help regulate attention.

Whether you could use a boost in focusing on your schoolwork or enhancing your mood and well-being, the solution might not be in your head but in your sneakers. "Exercise, no matter your age, is the single best thing you can do for every organ in your body, including your brain,"[32] says Allan Reiss, director of the Division of Interdisciplinary Brain Sciences at Stanford University School of Medicine. And those brain benefits include clearer thinking, better focus, and protection against mental troubles like stress, depression, and anxiety.

CHAPTER THREE

Get Ready to Move

Being active is a hallmark of youth. Some young people grow up playing sports and can't remember a time they weren't on a field, track, or court or in the pool competing on their own or as part of a team. For others, a martial arts center or dance studio was a home away from home. And many people can recall early days spent climbing trees, riding horses, or bouncing on a trampoline.

It was a trampoline injury that led Raunak Khosla to focus his sporting endeavors on swimming. In elementary school Khosla preferred football and lacrosse to swimming—a sport his older brother competed in year-round. But after breaking his arm in a trampoline accident, Khosla was sidelined from contact sports. Having competed in summer swim leagues as a child, Khosla returned to swimming in sixth grade. By the time he was in high school, he was being recruited by some of the top college swim programs in the country. He chose Princeton University, where in 2023 he earned the High Point Swimmer of the Ivy Championships—an award given to the Ivy League tournament's best swimmer.

And while the countless hours spent in the pool have taken him from Milton High School in Georgia to Princeton University and the National Collegiate Athletic Association Tournament three years in a row, the laps and competition have also served to support his mental health through the years. Swimming serves as a relaxing change of pace from the academic challenges of Princeton, while the classroom work and other responsibilities of college life help keep him from obsessing too much about swimming. "I think I've been lucky that I never see swimming as a chore, but rather as a great outlet," he told the college paper, the *Daily Princetonian*, in 2023. "It honestly helps me with the stress of school and vice-versa."[33]

Whatever activity you choose, you may find that it provides opportunities to release stress, expand your social circle, fuel your competitive fire, boost self-confidence, and much more. Deciding to become more physically active can lead to a lifetime of good mental and physical health. As you ponder what to do, keep in mind that what's right for you is all that matters. You may have friends, for example, who live, breathe, eat, and sleep cheerleading or basketball, but those activities hold no interest for you. Instead, you may love nothing more than spending hours in a dance studio or on mountain trails.

What's most important is that you move. Doing something is better than doing nothing. And if it's an activity you enjoy, you're more likely to stick with it. But if you do get bored with one activity or find it difficult to pursue for whatever reason, don't get discouraged. You can always find a new way to get your blood pumping and those endorphins flowing.

How Much Is Enough?

When committing to being more physically active, one of the first things you may wonder is just how much you need to do to feel better and maintain those mental health benefits. As with so many aspects of health and exercise, the answer depends on the individual. A couple of hours of physical activity a week may keep you energized and feeling great, while a friend of yours may need to work out for an hour a day just to shake off some stress and start to feel happy and hopeful.

A study of young people, published in the journal *Mental Health and Physical Activity* found that there was little difference in the rate of anxiety or depression between kids who exercised one to three days a week and those who exercised four to six days a week. Importantly, though, the researchers found that kids who didn't exercise at all were twice as likely as their active peers to have mental health problems.

Exercise isn't just about relieving stress and preventing mental health challenges; you need to move in order to stay physically healthy, too. The Centers for Disease Control and Prevention (CDC) recommends sixty minutes of physical activity per day for kids ages six to seventeen. The CDC adds that most of that time should be spent doing aerobic activities—things that get your heart beating faster—but if you can't do that every day, aim for at least three days a week of aerobic exercise. Muscle-strengthening activities such as push-ups, weight lifting, or climbing should also be done three days a week, as should bone-strengthening activities such as jumping, running, and resistance training.

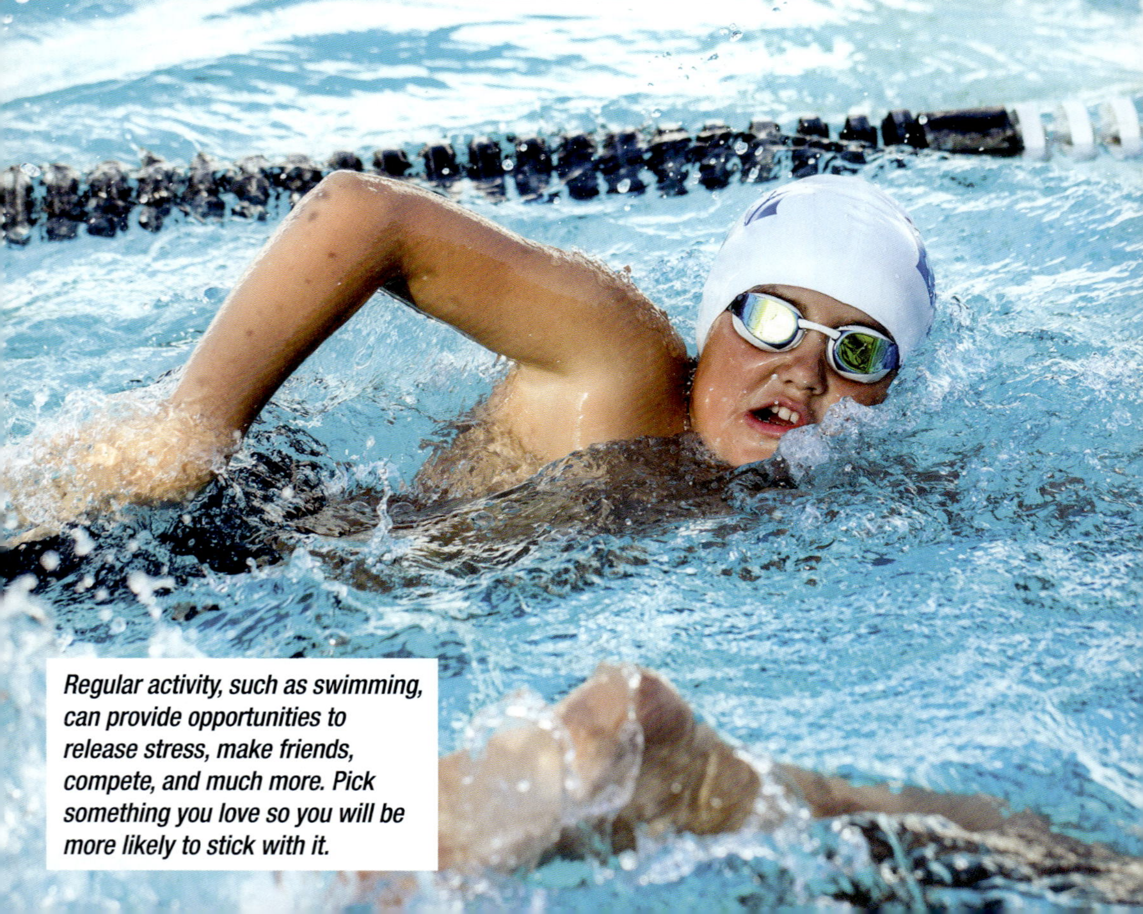

Regular activity, such as swimming, can provide opportunities to release stress, make friends, compete, and much more. Pick something you love so you will be more likely to stick with it.

Keep in mind that you don't have to get all your exercise and physical activity in during one long session. Breaking things up throughout the day can be just as healthy for your heart, lungs, and muscles. Short bursts of activity can also serve as helpful study breaks or opportunities to clear your mind if you've been doing homework for a while or dwelling on your problems. Good teachers also know that allowing their students to get up and move during the day keeps them more attentive and on task. Your mind needs a break now and then, and walking, running, or playing can make those breaks especially helpful.

Your optimal exercise time may also depend on how often and how intensely you feel discouraged or anxious. A 2018 study that appeared in the medical journal *The Lancet* notes that most people, on average, have a little more than three "poor mental health days" per month. Poor mental health was defined as having feelings of stress, depression, or other negative or troubling emotional concerns. But for people who exercise regularly, the number of poor mental health days dropped by more than 40 percent.

One other interesting finding from that study was that people can exercise "too much." The researchers found that three to five exercise or activity sessions of forty-five minutes or so each week provided the optimal mental health benefits. They also noted that after three hours of exercising, a person may start to develop worse mental symptoms compared with someone who doesn't exercise. While these numbers are averages and don't apply to every individual, they're worth keeping in mind as you develop your own routines.

Working out for hours at a time may be problematic because it suggests an underlying mental health issue, such as obsessive/compulsive disorder. Extra-long workouts may also lead to feelings of exhaustion, which can affect mood in a negative way. Of course, too much exercise can also put your physical health at risk. "If you exercise too much for weeks or months at a time, you put your body at risk of overtraining syndrome,"[34] says strength and conditioning specialist Alena Luciani in a 2022 article published in *Shape* magazine. Overtraining syndrome refers to muscle fibers not being able to repair themselves in between workouts and the body struggling in other ways to keep up with the demands of constant training. Overtraining may also lead to injuries that could keep you from exercising and gaining the many and varied benefits of physical activity.

How to Pick a Sport or Activity

A lot of factors go into choosing a sport, exercise routine, or other type of physical activity. You may want to do something that will build muscle, help you lose weight in a healthy way, allow you to play or work out with your friends, or be something you can do at home or in your neighborhood. You may prefer team sports to individual pursuits or vice versa.

Try to choose an activity that you enjoy and look forward to participating in on a regular basis. This will motivate you to keep moving. Activities that you dread or find stressful are not going to support your mental health. "The best exercise is the one that is actually done,"[35] says Andreas Heissel, a German researcher who led a large 2023 study demonstrating how physical activity helps lessen depression symptoms in young people.

One way to find a sport or activity that's right for you is to try a variety of things until you find the ones that keep you moving and motivated. Youth sport programs, including those in many schools, often emphasize the importance of specializing in one thing at the exclusion of other activities. But some schools are moving in a different direction. At Tuscarora High School in Maryland, kids of all skill levels are welcome to join school teams and are encouraged to sample several sports to find one or a few they like. "I'm from the mindset that you should do as many different sports as possible because you don't know what you're going to like,"[36] Tuscarora's athletics and facilities coordinator Chris O'Connor told NPR in 2023.

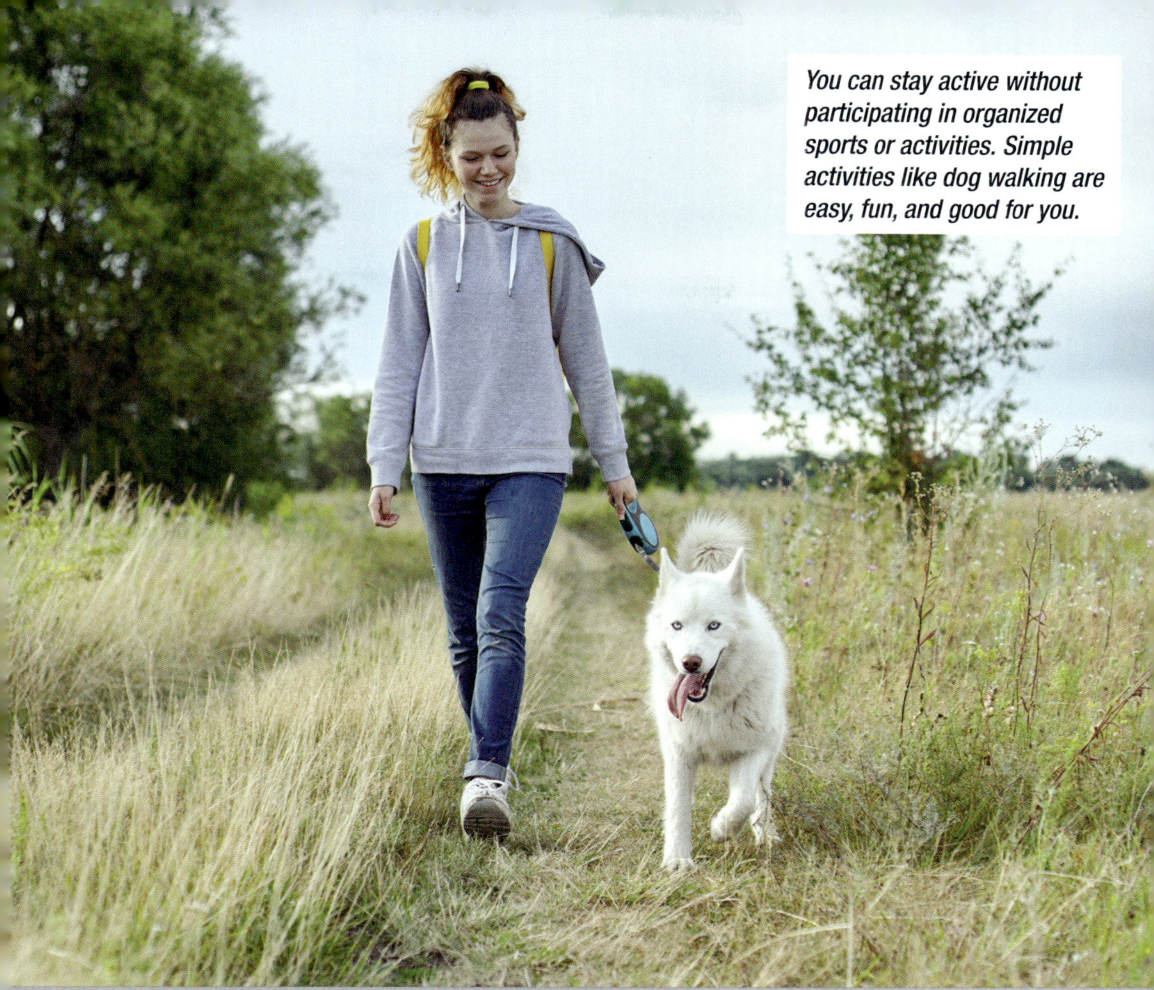

You can stay active without participating in organized sports or activities. Simple activities like dog walking are easy, fun, and good for you.

At the same time, Tuscarora's coaches acknowledge that sports aren't for everyone and that kids can be active in many other ways. That's a philosophy that is also gaining supporters as a response to youth sport programs that prioritize competition over fun. "I don't think forcing kids to play sports is a good idea," says Linda Flanagan, author of *Take Back the Game*, a book about the need for youth sport reform. "We have this distorted notion here about grit [a determined mindset]. Obviously grit is important. But I think we shouldn't make children stick with things just because it's a virtue to stick with things and who cares how miserable you are."[37]

If organized sports isn't your thing, you certainly have countless other options to stay active. Maybe you'll walk your dog one day, play tennis with your best friend the next day, and then go

Don't Forget to Take a Time-Out to Rest

Movement and exertion are great for body and mind, but you have to know when to take a break. If you exercise too much without allowing your muscles and the rest of your body a chance to recover, you risk injuries that can limit your ability to stay active. You also run the risk of burning out and losing interest in whatever sport or activity you had been enjoying. Everyone needs a mental break from school, work, and even friends and family members occasionally. And physical activity is no different, according to Cameron Apt, a certified strength and conditioning specialist with the University of Rochester Medical Center's Sports and Spine Rehabilitation Center. He says:

> There are some very clear signs that you are working out too much— besides physical fatigue, you typically will feel mentally lethargic, burned out, unenthusiastic. People who overdo it with workouts can even feel a sense of confusion. Whether you're an elite athlete, a weekend warrior, or someone who just wants to stay fit, it's important to listen to your body and respect it when it's telling you, "Enough."

Quoted in University of Rochester Medical Center, "Time Out: Why You Need a Break from Exercise," October 10, 2016. www.urmc.rochester.edu.

swimming, shoot baskets, go in-line skating, or lift weights on other days. Perhaps you will take a fitness class or find some exercise videos online. Consider activities you might never have thought about before, like horseback riding, fencing, ice-skating, paddleboarding, or martial arts. Theater classes often include dance instruction and stage combat training as well as movement and breathing exercises that can give you a workout.

Other factors to keep in mind when choosing a sport or exercise routine include the time needed from your weekly schedule, transportation arrangements and their potential cost, and the expense of lessons or equipment. Certain competitive sports, such as rowing or skiing, can cost thousands of dollars a year just to be a participant. A sport or activity that requires several hours of practice all or most days of the week may not fit with your schedule or that of your family. It's important to talk about these things with your parents or guardians, especially if you're relying on them to help pay for it or get you to and from practices and competitions.

You should also view activities for how they line up with what you enjoy and with what you want to get out of those activities. Team sports offer a social benefit that individual sports do not. You might be more comfortable on a playing field where victory or defeat is a shared responsibility. However, if you're the kind of person who wants to be alone in the spotlight and succeed or fail on your own—as with tennis, golf, figure skating, swimming, martial arts, or other individual sports—then look into those activities. Think about what you truly want and why, and then make your decision.

Don't assume that an activity will be too expensive or inconvenient for your family without first talking about it. Your parents may be just as enthusiastic as you are when it comes to exploring a new activity. And if money or scheduling is a challenge, look around for alternatives. Maybe there's a lower-cost program in your community, or perhaps you have a friend whose family can share in the transportation responsibility.

The Benefits of Certain Activities

Cost, scheduling, and your own personal interests are just some of the things to consider when selecting a sport or activity. Researchers have found that certain sports and exercise regimens offer their own distinct advantages. For example, team sports help foster friendships and ease social anxiety. Being part of a team also enhances feelings of belonging, responsibility, and a sense of purpose. "We know that kids benefit from social interactions. They can make friends on teams. They generally, hopefully, have a good time and these factors might sort of protect them from any mental health challenges or difficulties they might experience,"[38] says Matt Hoffmann, a professor of kinesiology at California State University, Fullerton. He is also the author of a 2022 study that suggests kids who play team sports tend to have fewer mental health struggles than their peers who don't participate in sports.

Sports that build or tone muscles, such as resistance training and climbing, can build confidence and self-esteem. Dancing can also boost your confidence and ease social anxiety. And the unique nature of swimming and the therapeutic nature of being in water have their own rewards. "Swimming alleviates stress and encourages relaxation and creativity as the feeling of water moving over our body creates a massage-like sensation," says Hana Patel, a physician and mental health coach in England. "It helps release pent-up tension and also makes us more mindful of our surroundings."[39]

Not surprisingly, exercises and activities that contain an element of mindfulness and relaxation can be particularly helpful

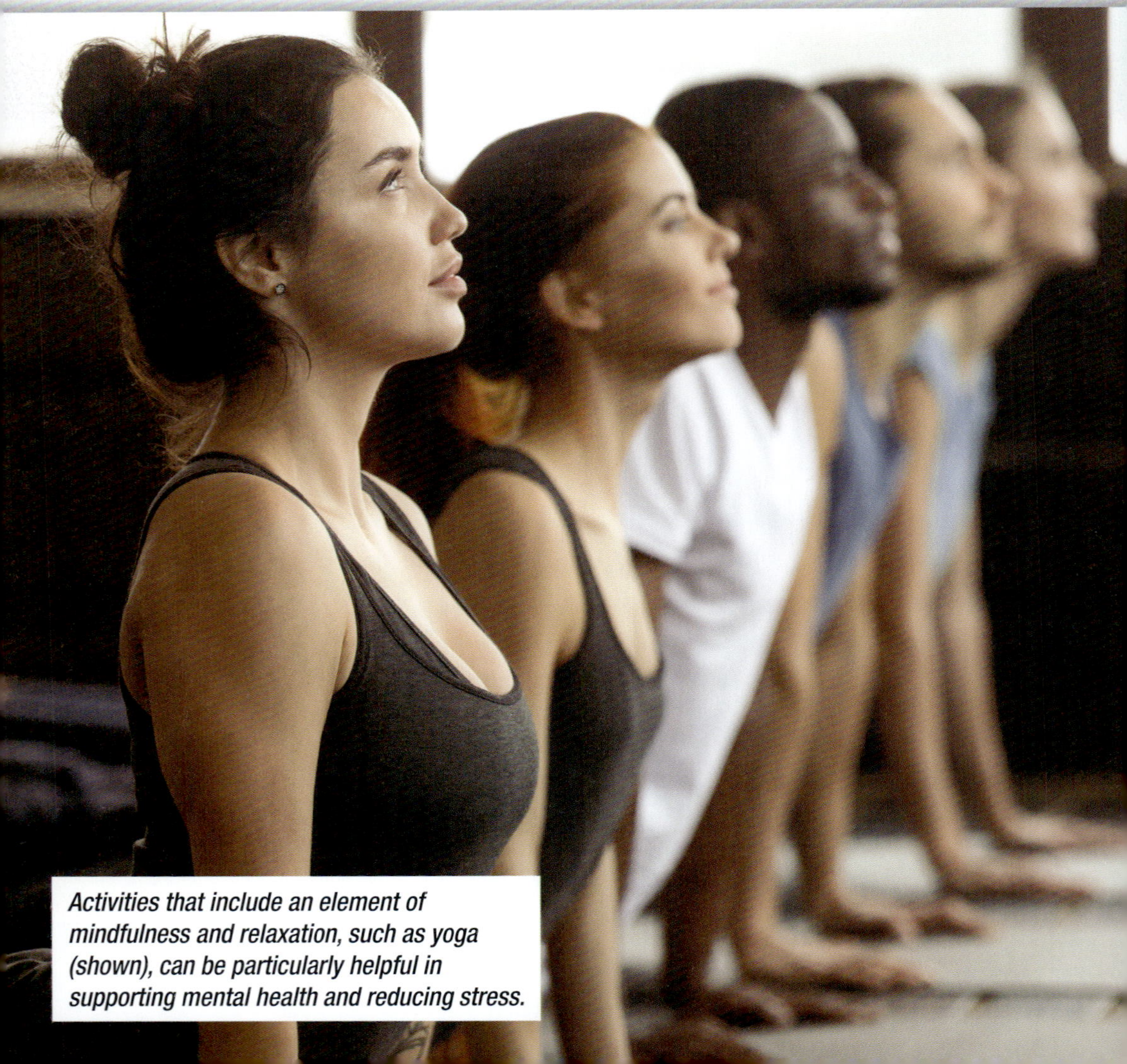

Activities that include an element of mindfulness and relaxation, such as yoga (shown), can be particularly helpful in supporting mental health and reducing stress.

An Activity for Life

While you might be looking for an activity to occupy your time right now, keep in mind that you may be starting on a lifelong journey with your new sport or pastime. Golf, tennis, swimming, cycling—the list goes on of sports enjoyed by kids and seniors alike. And you don't know where a new activity will take you or how it might inspire you. Leigha Porter started dancing as a little girl in Lafayette, Indiana. Back then it was just something fun to do with her friends. But as she got older and committed herself to dance, she wound up performing in theaters across the country. As an adult, the dancer became a creator, returning to Lafayette and founding Parc Village, a community arts program that welcomes new generations of young artists. "I wanted to put something in a community that was easily accessible to everyone," Porter said in an interview with KATC News. "I want people to be introduced to different visual artists, just bringing that realness and culture and truly staying true to who I am. I want to do what I can do for my community."

Quoted in Katie Lopez, "Women's History Month: Leigha Porter," KATC News, March 17, 2023. www.katc.com.

in supporting mental health and reducing stress. Few exercises are as aligned with mental and physical health as yoga. Studies have shown that yoga can often help people deal with symptoms related to post-traumatic stress disorder and obsessive-compulsive disorder. It can also help with everyday stress and self-confidence. "A child's yoga practice is a rare opportunity to experience play and focus without worrying about being wrong,"[40] says Shana Meyerson, who teaches yoga to kids in Southern California.

Alexandra De Collibus, a Massachusetts yoga instructor who teaches youth classes, adds that the calming, meditative aspects of yoga can help people find inner peace. "Since the modern world moves very, very fast for children, it's not long before they feel all kinds of pressure (personal, parental, social) to keep up with everyone around them," she says. "Yoga functions as a release valve that

> "A child's yoga practice is a rare opportunity to experience play and focus without worrying about being wrong."[40]
>
> —Shana Meyerson, yoga instructor

alleviates pressure and as a foundation to nurture and develop a resilient and resourceful body, mind, and spirit."[41] And the physical fitness component of yoga, with its emphasis on flexibility and strength, can be a nice complement for keeping in shape for activities ranging from baseball and basketball to cheerleading, dance, and running.

Whatever gets you moving, the key is to do the exercise or play the sport that's best for you. Find activities that are fun but challenging so you won't get bored or frustrated—neither of which will help your mental health.

CHAPTER FOUR

Overcoming Obstacles to Physical Activity

You know that exercise and physical activity will give you energy, strength, and stamina, as well as boost your mental health. But you may have reasons why you're not more active. Perhaps you have physical limitations that make it difficult to exercise. Or maybe you've been sedentary for so long that you're unsure how to get more physical activity into your routine. And if you're struggling with depression, it can be difficult to motivate yourself to exercise or engage in physical activity at all.

Whatever may be in your way, there are means to overcome or sidestep such obstacles. The first step is to be realistic about exercising, regardless of what may be holding you back, says Nicholas Forand, an assistant professor of psychiatry at Zucker School of Medicine at Hofstra/Northwell Health in New York. "People often say they're going to wake up at 5:30 and go to the gym when there's a zero percent chance that that's actually going to happen. You set yourself up to fail," he says. "Set realistic expectations for yourself."[42]

It may take you a few tries to establish a consistent exercise regimen, and that's okay. If your goal was to ramp up your activity level starting on the weekend and those days fly by without much change, that's okay. Focus on starting things off the following weekend or during the week. There's nothing special about a day on a calendar. Plenty of New Year's resolutions don't begin on January 1. Being more physically active is for your health and well-being, so what you do and when you do it are up to you.

Sometimes, committing to a more active lifestyle requires a new way of thinking and being more resourceful with what you have to work with. In other cases you may need to get some therapy or recruit friends or family members to get you up and moving.

Overcoming Low Mood and Low Energy

One of the most common symptoms of depression—even mild depression—is a lack of motivation or energy to exercise or do much physical activity at all. The situation is made worse when depression brings on body aches, sleep problems, and an increased perception of pain. No one wants to exercise when they're not feeling good. But physical symptoms brought on by depression are unfortunate because regular physical activity has been shown to reduce depressive symptoms.

One way to overcome depression's grip on your motivation is to try for short, manageable bursts of activity. The idea of getting up and working out for half an hour or an hour may seem daunting, even if you don't have severe depression. Instead, assistant professor of psychiatry Michael Craig Miller suggests, break down your big exercise goal into a few minutes here and there. "Start with five minutes a day of walking or any activity you enjoy," he says. "Soon, five minutes of activity will become 10, and 10 will become 15."[43]

And don't feel that your activity choice must be a brisk walk, a sport, or a workout in a fitness center. Dancing to music alone in your room or dancing while you vacuum or do other chores can be a great workout. Jump rope at home. Take your dog for

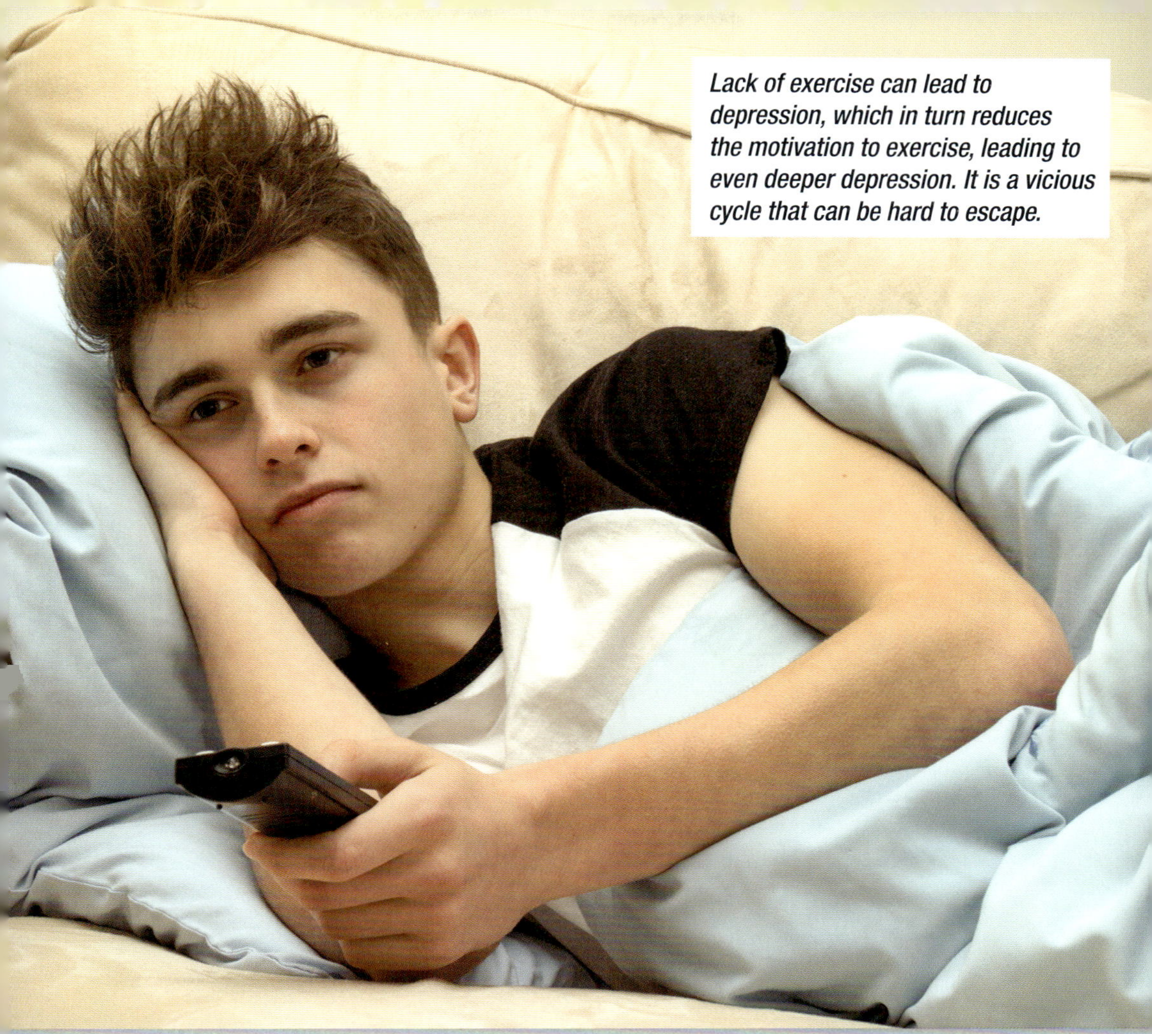

an extra-long walk or run, or volunteer to do so for a neighbor. "The thing is, there are so many ways to move your body," says neuroscientist and New York University professor Wendy Suzuki. "It's hard to get someone who does not exercise to move regularly. Once you get over the hump, you can start to be much more mindful and see and feel the immediate effects of exercise—you are literally changing your brain."[44]

If you are truly unable to summon the energy and motivation to exercise or change your usual routine, talk with a doctor or therapist. The struggle to get up and get moving is not a character flaw or a sign of weakness. It's common, but it's manageable.

> **"The thing is, there are so many ways to move your body."[44]**
>
> —Wendy Suzuki, neuroscientist and New York University professor

Explore Alternatives

Exercises like walking or playing basketball or soccer at a nearby park can be relatively inexpensive and flexible enough to fit into most any schedule. But sometimes what you want to do can't be so easily accomplished. You may need to work part-time after school, which makes playing on a school sports team difficult. Joining a fitness center can be expensive. You may not have enough friends who want to play baseball or softball.

When these kinds of hurdles appear in front of you, think about how you can get around them. If buying a set of weights for your home isn't feasible and joining a gym isn't either, see about getting resistance bands. You find these supersized rubber bands online or in sporting goods stores or even big department stores for a lot less money than a set of dumbbells and barbells.

You may also find used low-cost sports equipment online, at garage sales, or at resale stores. If you don't mind slightly used hockey sticks, golf clubs, baseball gloves, or tennis rackets, these items may be the ticket.

If after-school sports aren't an option, look around your community for sports programs that take place on the weekends or have evening schedules. Your local YMCA or other nonprofit fitness and sports organizations usually offer leagues throughout the year. Many of these programs also offer scholarships or reduced rates if finances are a challenge. Just ask one of the organizers.

Volunteering to help coach in a rec league or other sports program is another option. Coaching allows you to get out and play while also helping others. Many high schools require a certain number of volunteer hours to graduate, and college and scholarship programs are also looking at community service as part of a well-rounded high school experience.

Many programs for children with disabilities are also frequently looking for young volunteers to help. Programs such as the Special Olympics and the Miracle League not only allow you to become more active for your own mental health, they also let you make a big difference in the lives of others. University of Wisconsin

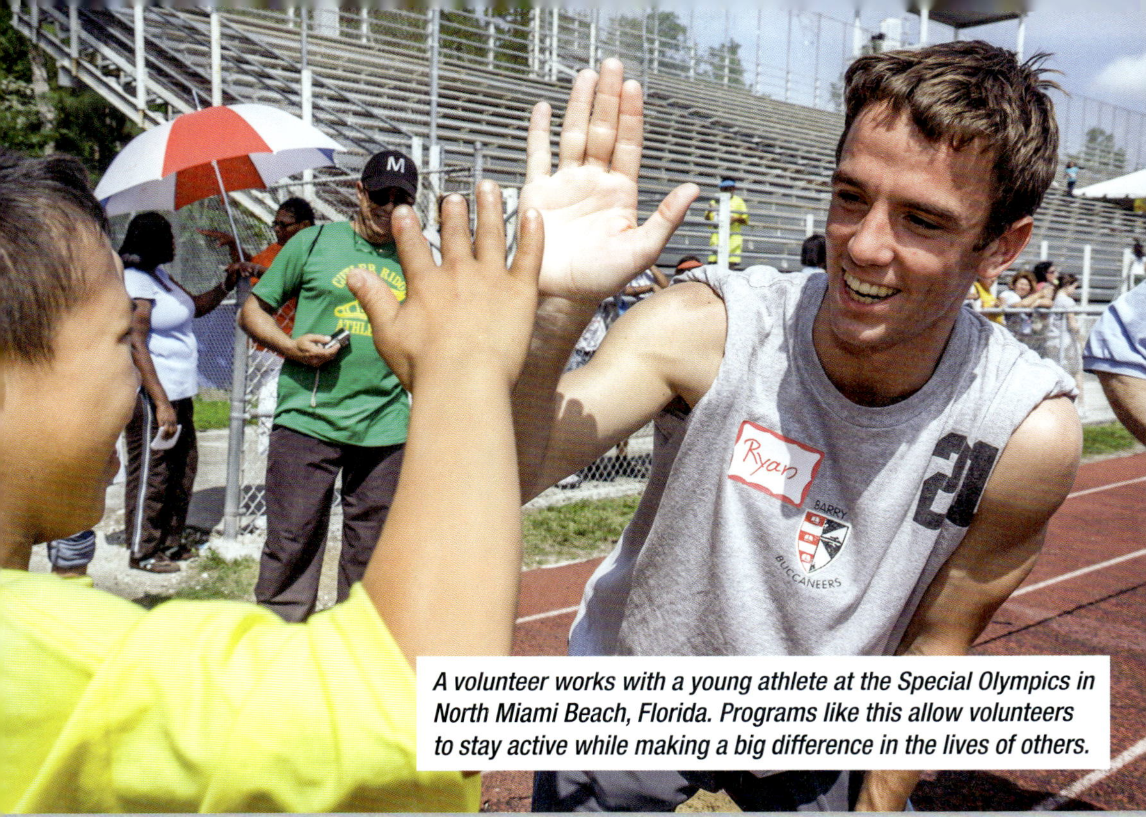

A volunteer works with a young athlete at the Special Olympics in North Miami Beach, Florida. Programs like this allow volunteers to stay active while making a big difference in the lives of others.

freshman swimmer Abby Wanezek joined several other athletes in the summer of 2023 to assist with Miracle League baseball games in Madison. "Just seeing the reaction on the kids' faces, seeing how much fun they're having and the impact that it's creating, I really want this to be a life-lasting memory," she said. "I hope it is. It feels great to be out with these kids. I didn't know something like this would feel this way. The reward I feel—how happy I'm feeling inside—is the highlight of my week."[45]

Change of Habit

You may have heard the expression that people are "creatures of habit," meaning we tend to get into a routine of doing the same thing the same way. Habits and routines aren't necessarily bad. If you do your homework right after dinner every night instead of right after school, and all your work gets done with that approach, then that could be considered a good habit worth continuing. But if waiting until the evening to do your homework means you're too tired to concentrate well or you're easily distracted by friends texting you, then you may need to rethink your homework habits.

Routines can also be thought of in terms of physics. One of Newton's laws of motion says that an object in motion remains in motion at constant speed and moving in a straight line unless acted on by another force. In other words, things will usually keep going along without changing until something forces a change. If your daily routine doesn't include time for physical activity, then you may need to create that force to change your direction. Habits are hard to break, but if shaking up your routine means you get more exercise, then you should consider finding some way to be that "other force" in your own life.

During the school day it can be difficult to get in as much physical activity as you'd like, since most of your time is spent sitting in class. But when you get chances to move around at school, take advantage of them. And when you're home or somewhere with a more relaxed schedule, form a new habit of frequently getting up from your computer or other stationary position and walking, stretching, or moving in some way.

Dr. Erin Michos, an associate professor of medicine at Johns Hopkins University School of Medicine, explains that the lasting benefits of physical activity come from moving consistently throughout the day, every day, rather than from intensive but just occasional workouts. Michos says:

> You don't have to replace sitting with time at the gym. There's benefit to light activity during the day. For every 20 minutes of sitting, try to stand for eight minutes and move around for two minutes. I recommend everybody track their steps, with a fitness tracker, your phone or a simple pedometer. We usually recommend a target of 10,000 steps a day. But if you're very sedentary, any improvement will be beneficial. If you only get 2,000 steps a day, try to aim for 4,000. Take baby steps. It doesn't have to be vigorous. Just stand up and move your muscles.[46]

A First Time for Everything

One common obstacle to regular exercise or athletic participation is the belief that you can't compete with others, especially if you're new to the sport or activity. Feeling self-conscious about how much weight you can lift, how fast you can run, or how well you can play a particular sport shouldn't keep you from joining in. One strategy that can help is to work out or play with a friend who won't judge you or your abilities. You can also find a recreational sports league where there are plenty of other beginners and the atmosphere is oriented toward having fun over winning. And remember that most people working out or otherwise being active are focused on themselves and not on anyone else. "If you're on a ski slope, most people aren't looking for the beginners, to laugh at them and evaluate them," says Keith Rollag, an organizational behavior researcher and professor at Babson College. "They're just going down the mountain." And the more experienced people around you were beginners once and may be willing to help you learn, especially if you happily acknowledge your inexperience and ask nicely for assistance.

Quoted in Cari Romm, "A Psychologist Explains How to Conquer Your Fear of Trying New Things," The Cut, January 9, 2018. www.thecut.com.

If you used to be more physically active, think about your old habits and how you fit activity into your schedule. The secret for you may be to rekindle an old habit, because your brain's old neural pathways that guided your thoughts and behaviors are still there ready to serve. Creating new neural pathways for new habits can be tougher than relying on established ones, says neuropsychologist Amy Serin, chief science office of the TouchPoint Solution health care tech company. "So if you used to do a kickboxing workout regularly, for example, start with that because the habit can be reactivated easier than starting something totally new. Use your neural networks to your advantage,"[47] she says.

Stick to a Schedule

Once you've embarked on your new healthy habit, you may need to establish a schedule to keep you from slipping back into a sedentary routine. One of the advantages of organized sports, extracurricular activities, dance lessons, or other structured programs is that they provide a regular schedule that you can incorporate into your school and home routines. Some kids need more structured activities to stay focused and stick with the activity. Others can be active without set practices and events on the calendar. Think about what works best for you and make your choices accordingly.

If you already have a busy schedule with school, extracurricular activities, homework, family obligations, and other time-consuming responsibilities, look for ways to mix physical activity into your day in small bursts. Maybe your daily routine allows for a quick workout between homework and dinner or a sports practice right after school. You may be best served with an early morning yoga session before school, free time after school, and a walk around your neighborhood after dinner. Being busy shouldn't be a reason to skip exercise altogether. And on days when you have more flexibility or free time, consider doing a little extra.

As you add more physical activity to your daily or weekly schedule, be aware of how this change is affecting your mental health. As much as exercise can be helpful, taking on too much at one time can have the opposite effect and make you more stressed out. If you're unsure how to manage your schedule, talk with your parents or other adults about strategies to manage it all, or consider dropping one activity to make room for a new one.

Burnout

Unfortunately, stress can accompany sports and other activities. Sometimes reluctance to participate in a sport or exercise routine is simply a response to the activity itself. You may have played a particular sport for a long time and no longer find it fun or rewarding. This is especially common among athletes who focus on one sport and play it year-round.

To recognize and avoid burnout, ask yourself whether you still enjoy the activity and want to continue with it. Maybe you just need a break for a while, or perhaps you need to assess whether an activity is too demanding. If you're on a highly competitive club soccer team, for example, you may want to step back and find a recreational program that demands less of your time but still allows you to play a sport you love. You might benefit from playing a mix of sports throughout the year. "Children who aren't spending all their time on one activity are at lower risk for burnout,"[48] says Miriam Rowan, a psychologist with the Boston Children's Hospital Female Athlete Program.

It's also important to ask yourself whether you are playing a sport or participating in dance or other activity because it's what you want or because you think it's what your parents want or what you feel you must do to land a college scholarship. Burnout can be a self-induced problem, brought on by an intense effort to be the best or the difficulty of separating your athletic performance from who you are as a person. In California, Fountain Valley High School senior and former varsity swimmer Jovana Hester told the *Los Angeles Times* in the fall of 2021 that the

> "Children who aren't spending all their time on one activity are at lower risk for burnout."[48]
>
> —Miriam Rowan, psychologist with Boston Children's Hospital Female Athlete Program

pressure she put on herself to improve her times and the pressure she felt from her parents and coaches triggered a great deal of anxiety and burnout. She eventually quit the sport. "Toward the end, I started to experience that heavy level of anxiety that started to become debilitating, or I couldn't really focus on my practices and I couldn't focus on anything other than swimming while outside of swim,"[49] Hester said.

Young people tend to be especially self-critical, whether it's in sports, academics, the arts, or their interactions with others. "Some athletes tend to be overly critical of themselves and their athletic skills. They're unable to separate their athletic development from whether they win or lose," says Kelsey Griffith, mental skills specialist with the Micheli Center for Sports Injury Prevention

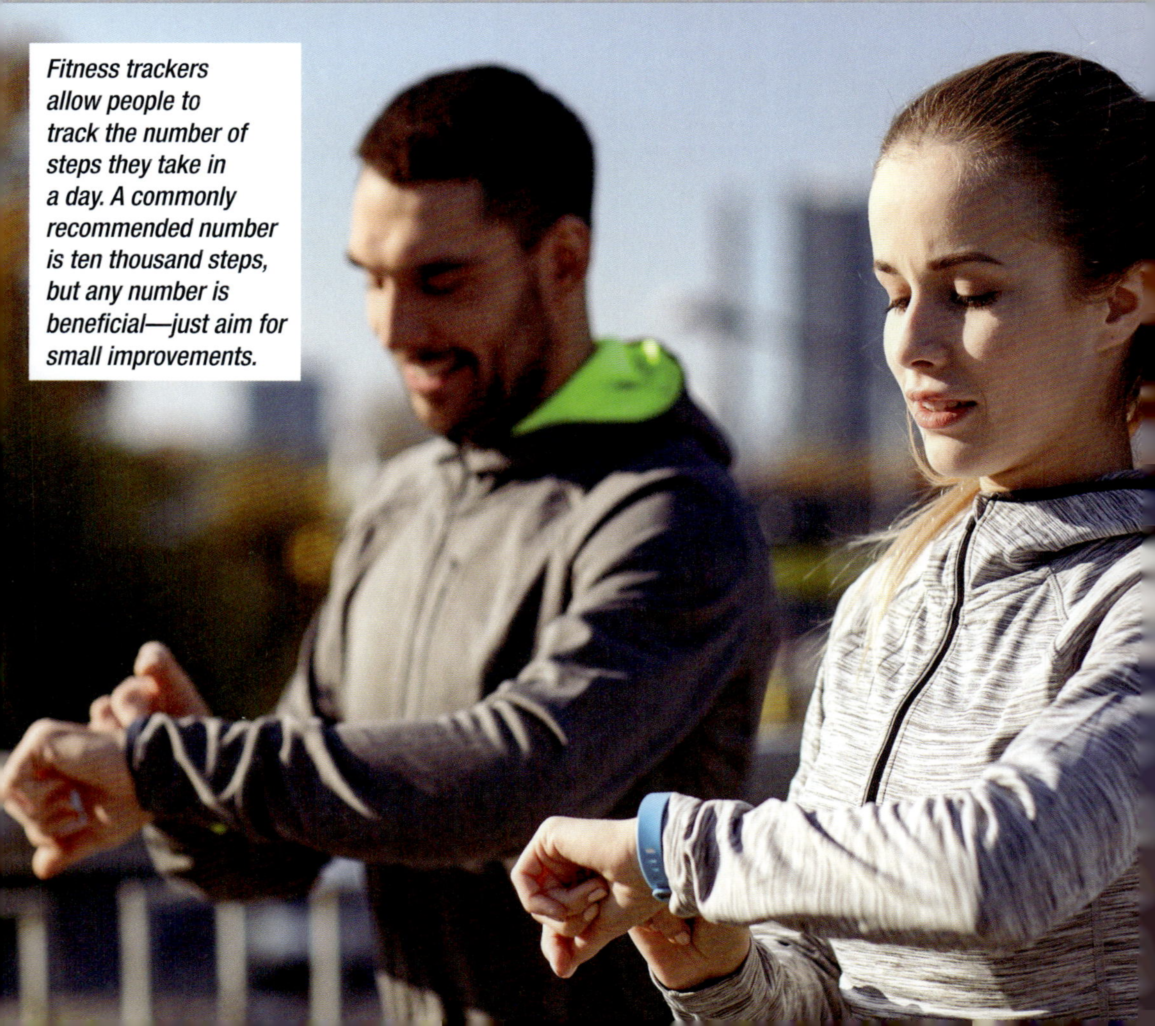

Fitness trackers allow people to track the number of steps they take in a day. A commonly recommended number is ten thousand steps, but any number is beneficial—just aim for small improvements.

in Massachusetts. "No matter how well they're performing, they never feel like they're good enough."[50]

Your mental health and feelings about a sport are far more important than personal bests, wins, and losses. If you're feeling overwhelmed, anxious, or otherwise uncomfortable about your sport or activity, sharing your concerns with your coaches, instructors, and parents may be the first step in finding a new way to approach your sport or find a new activity altogether. Remember that "play" is the main part of playing a sport.

Dealing with a Disability

For some kids, play can also require a lot of work and effort. Having physical limitations due to a chronic medical condition or disability isn't your fault, and it can present real challenges to becoming more active. For example, having a visual impairment or requiring a wheelchair or walker to get around means you must make other considerations or seek accommodations that other kids don't need. But in recent years, exercise experts, physical therapists, sports coaches, and others have developed a range of exercises and athletic options for people who need to make certain adaptations to their activities or choose pursuits that fit with their needs and abilities.

Water-based exercises, chair yoga, adaptive athletic equipment (like that used in the Paralympics and Special Olympics), and other tools can help just about anyone become more active. Think about sports and activities you've seen in person, online, or on television. You may be surprised to learn that there are leagues and organizations ready to provide those same opportunities to young people in your community.

Canadian athlete, model, and motivational speaker Allison Lang was born without the lower portion of her left leg. She has been active her entire life, even earning a spot on the Canadian Women's Sitting Volleyball Team and competing around the world. She told Yahoo! Life in 2022:

It's been an amazing experience to work with this amazing group of women. We are so connected, we're fearless, we're fit, and we are working to get sitting volleyball on the map. Our sport has grown so much and I'm really proud of what we have accomplished, and what we will accomplish in the future. We're trying to show people that even though you may be disabled, you can still be a national athlete. You can still represent your country.[51]

Just Move

While more physical activity is usually better than less, and though certain activities may offer more mental health benefits than others, the most important thing to remember is just to move. Move throughout the day. Move most (if not all) days of the week. And if you need help getting motivated or with the activities themselves, ask for some assistance. You don't have to play on a sports team or join a gym or climb mountains. Just move and remember that you and your well-being matter. And if the activities you choose aren't helping you feel better, you have a whole world of options just waiting to be explored.

SOURCE NOTES

Introduction: Stay Active, Feel Better

1. Katharina Star, "The Mental Health Benefits of Physical Exercise," Verywell Mind, January 3, 2023. www.verywellmind.com.
2. Quoted in Donna Whitehead, "Taunton Teens to Fellow Students: 'It's OK Not to Be OK,'" *Taunton (MA) Gazette*, May 27, 2022. www.tauntongazette.com.
3. Jeremy Whitworth, "Six Mental Health Benefits of Exercise in Teens," Trails Carolina, March 23, 2023. https://trailscarolina.com.
4. Quoted in Harvard Medical School, "Exercise Is an All-Natural Treatment to Fight Depression," February 2, 2021. www.health.harvard.edu.

Chapter One: The Mind–Body Connection

5. Quoted in Melissa Eichman, "Bay Area Teen Dances for Mental Health Awareness," Bay News 9, April 17, 2023. www.baynews9.com.
6. David J. Linden, "The Truth Behind 'Runner's High' and Other Mental Benefits of Running," Johns Hopkins Medicine, 2023. www.hopkinsmedicine.org.
7. Quoted in UNC Health Talk, "The Power of Laughter for Your Health," June 9, 2020. https://healthtalkunchealthcare.org.
8. Quoted in Kathiann Kowalski, "Too Much Sitting Could Hurt Your Mental Health," Science News Explores, April 15, 2021. www.snexplores.org.
9. Quoted in Iowa State University, "Sitting More Linked to Feelings of Depression, Anxiety," ScienceDaily. November 8, 2021. www.sciencedaily.com.
10. Quoted in Matthew Solan, "The Book of Neurogenesis," Harvard Medical School, August 1, 2021. www.health.harvard.edu.
11. Quoted in Harvard Medical School, "Exercise Is an All-Natural Treatment to Fight Depression."
12. Quoted in *Oregon Health News Blog*, "How Exercise Impacts Your Brain," September 8, 2022. https://covidblog.oregon.gov.
13. Justin Rhodes, "Why Is It That I Seem to Think Better When I Walk or Exercise?," *Scientific American*, July 1, 2013. www.scientificamerican.com.
14. Quoted in Stephen Schramm, "Exercise Your Body to Keep Your Mind Healthy," Duke Today, June 12, 2023. https://today.duke.edu.

15. Quoted in Mercey Livingston, "Need Motivation? 4 Unexpected Benefits for Your Happiness," CNET, March 29, 2023. www.cnet.com.

16. Quoted in Johns Hopkins Medicine, "Exercising for Better Sleep," 2023. www.hopkinsmedicine.org.

17. Quoted in Johns Hopkins Medicine, "Exercising for Better Sleep."

18. Quoted in University of South Australia, "Sleep Keeps Teens on Track for Good Mental Health," February 10, 2021. www.unisa.edu.au.

Chapter Two: Movement and Mental Health

19. Quoted in Piper Winton, "Riverside Soccer Improves Athletes' Mental Health During COVID-19 Pandemic," *Pirate's Hook*, November 8, 2021. https://thepirateshook.com.

20. Quoted in Winton, "Riverside Soccer Improves Athletes' Mental Health During COVID-19 Pandemic."

21. Quoted in Perri Klass, "The Benefits of Exercise for Children's Mental Health," *New York Times*, March 2, 2020. www.nytimes.com.

22. Quoted in Gretchen Reynolds, "The Best Treatment for Depression Could Be Exercise," *Washington Post*, March 15, 2023. www.washingtonpost.com.

23. Quoted in Jade Scipioni, "Lindsey Vonn Spent Her 19-Year Career Battling Depression—Here Are the Tactics She Used to Stay at the Top," CNBC. November 19, 2021. www.cnbc.com.

24. Emma Nushi, "How Being an Athlete Saved My Mental Health During the Pandemic," *The Cuestonian*, November 5, 2020. www.cuestonian.com.

25. Quoted in Nikki Campo, "Why Bicycling Might Keep Your Kid's Mental Health in High Gear," National Geographic, September 6, 2022. www.nationalgeographic.com.

26. Quoted in Sarah Elizabeth Richards, "7 Benefits of Strength Training That Go Beyond Building Muscle," NBC News, February 8, 2018. www.nbcnews.com.

27. Quoted in Lisa Rapaport, "Yes, Counting Steps Might Make You Healthier," Reuters, June 25, 2019. www.reuters.com.

28. Quoted in Melanie Radzicki McManus, "How to Help Your Teen Get Moving," CNN, September 22, 2022. www.cnn.com.

29. Quoted in Elea Abisamra, "Socializing Now Is Crucial for Longevity and Mental Health," *Collegiate Times*. October 17, 2022. www.collegiatetimes.com.

30. Quoted in Charlotte Nguyen, "Mental Health in Student Athletes," Slick, May 31, 2023. https://hbslick.com.

31. Quoted in John Ratey, "The ADHD Exercise Solution," *ADDitude*, February 8, 2023. www.additudemag.com.

32. Quoted in Campo, "Why Bicycling Might Keep Your Kid's Mental Health in High Gear."

Chapter Three: Get Ready to Move

33. Quoted in Hayk Yengibaryan, "From the Pool to the Podium: The Rise of Rank Khosla," *Daily Princetonian*, March 22, 2023. www.dailyprincetonian.com.
34. Quoted in Gabrielle Kassel, "How Much Exercise Is Too Much?," *Shape*, May 13, 2022. www.shape.com.
35. Quoted in Reynolds, "The Best Treatment for Depression Could Be Exercise."
36. Quoted in Selena Simmons-Duffin, "Kids Can't All Be Star Athletes. Here's How Schools Can Welcome More Students to Play," NPR, June 7, 2023. www.npr.org.
37. Quoted in Selna Simmons-Duffin, "Kids Can't All Be Star Athletes."
38. Quoted in Megan Calongne, "Study Shows Link Between Kid Team Sports and Mental Health," KBTX News, June 7, 2022. www.kbtx .com.
39. Quoted in Caitlin Tilley, "Run to Think Clearly, Dance to Shake Off Anxiety and Swim to Calm Nerves: How Different Exercises Improve Your Mental Health," *Daily Mail* (London), October 25, 2022. www .dailymail.co.uk.
40. Quoted in Nicole Harris, "11 Benefits of Yoga for Kids," *Parents*, May 20, 2023. www.parents.com.
41. Quoted in Harris, "11 Benefits of Yoga for Kids."

Chapter Four: Overcoming Obstacles to Physical Activity

42. Quoted in Rajul Punjabi, "How to Get Yourself to Exercise If You're Depressed," *Vice*, May 23, 2018. www.vice.com.
43. Quoted in Harvard Medical School, "Exercise Is an All-Natural Treatment to Fight Depression."
44. Quoted in Deborah Farmer Kris, "How Movement and Exercise Help Kids Learn," KQED, May 21, 2019. www.kqed.org.
45. Quoted in Andy Baggot, "Miracle League Partnership Is Life Changing, for All Involved," University of Wisconsin, July 27, 2023. https:// uwbadgers.com.
46. Erin Michos, "Sitting Disease: How a Sedentary Lifestyle Affects Heart Health," Johns Hopkins Medicine, 2023. www.hopkins medicine.org.
47. Quoted in Punjabi, "How to Get Yourself to Exercise If You're Depressed."

48. Quoted in Boston Children's Hospital, "Keeping Sports Fun: Preventing Burnout in Young Athletes," September 15, 2022. https://answers.childrenshospital.org.
49. Quoted in Reese Meister, "Athletes Bring Mental Health to the Forefront of Conversation in Sports," *Los Angeles Times*, November 9, 2021. https://highschool.latimes.com.
50. Quoted in Boston Children's Hospital, "Keeping Sports Fun."
51. Quoted in Julia Ranney, "Canadian Amputee Allison Lang on Modelling, Fitness and Finding Self-Confidence," Yahoo! Life, August 23, 2022. https://ca.style.yahoo.com.

ORGANIZATIONS AND WEBSITES

Centers for Disease Control and Prevention
www.cdc.gov/healthyschools/physicalactivity/guidelines.htm
The site includes the highlights from the *Physical Activity Guidelines for Americans*, as well as a link to the entire publication. In addition to spelling out recommendations for daily and weekly exercise goals, the site includes important information about how physical activity supports academic performance, attention, and better mental health.

Mental Health Literacy
https://mentalhealthliteracy.org
This organization is a resource for teens as well as family members, teachers, counselors, and health professionals interested in promoting good mental health. There is information about various mental health challenges, how to improve your sleep, and many other subjects presented in accessible, easy-to-understand language.

National Institute of Mental Health (NIMH)
www.nimh.nih.gov/news/science-news/science-news-about-children-and-adolescents
The "Science News About Children and Adolescents" section of the NIMH website includes warning signs of a mental health or behavioral disorder, as well as advice for you or someone you know who might need help. You can also find links to many mental health topics and news articles covering issues ranging from the science of the brain to how mental health disorders are diagnosed and treated.

Nemours TeensHealth
https://kidshealth.org/en/teens/exercise-wise.html
On this site you can learn how exercise is good for every part of the body as well as for your mental health. There is information on aerobic exercise, strength training, and flexibility and helpful advice to stick with your exercise routine.

Teen Health Matters
https://teenhealthmatters.org
You can find information here about stress management, mental health, and physical health. Topics include choosing healthy foods, ways to stay active, warning signs of mental illness, and many more. There are also links to podcasts and videos featuring experts as well as young people discussing a wide range of mental and physical health topics.

FOR FURTHER RESEARCH

Books

Jennie Marie Battisin, *Mindfulness for Teens in 10 Minutes a Day*. Emeryville, CA: Rockridge, 2019.

Al Desetta, *Healthy Living for Teens: Inspiring Advice on Diet, Exercise, and Handling Stress*. New York: Sky Pony, 2021.

Brandi Matz, *Anxiety Relief Journal for Teens*. Emeryville, CA: Rockridge, 2021.

Paula Nagel, *The Mental Health and Wellbeing Workout for Teens*. London: Jessica Kingsley, 2019.

Varuna Shingle and Ken Spillman, *More than I Am: Yoga Wisdom for 21st Century Teens*. New Delhi, India: HarperCollins India, 2023.

Internet Sources

Centers for Disease Control and Prevention, "Physical Activity Guidelines for School-Aged Children and Adolescents," 2023. www.cdc.gov.

Harvard Medical School, "More Evidence That Exercise Can Boost Mood," May 1, 2019. www.health.harvard.edu.

Perri Klass, "The Benefits of Exercise for Children's Mental Health," *New York Times*, March 2, 2020. www.nytimes.com.

National Institute of Mental Health, "Teen Depression: More than Just Moodiness," 2023. www.nimh.nih.gov.

University of Rochester Medical Center, "Exercise and Teenagers," 2023. www.urmc.rochester.edu.

Jeremy Whitworth, "Six Mental Health Benefits of Exercise in Teens," Trails Carolina, March 23, 2023. https://trailscarolina.com.

PICTURE CREDITS

Cover: Shutterstock.com

 6: Lopolo/Shutterstock.com

10: DavideAngelini/Shutterstock.com

13: Fizkes/Shutterstock.com

17: New Africa/Shutterstock.com

21: PeopleImages.com-Yuri A/Shutterstock.com

22: Action Plus Sports Images/Alamy Stock Photo

28: Simonkr/Shutterstock.com

32: Karlnoppe/Shutterstock.com

35: VH-Studio/Shutterstock.com

38: Fizkes/Shutterstock.com

43: Ben Gingell/Shutterstock.com

45: Jeff Isaac Greenberg 13+/Alamy Stock Photo

50: Ground Picture/Shutterstock.com

ABOUT THE AUTHOR

After graduating from the University of Oregon, James Roland became a newspaper reporter, primarily focused on education. He later became a magazine writer and editor, as well as an author of more than a dozen books. He and his wife, Heidi, have three children, Chris, Alexa, and Carson.